Also by Susan Q. Knittle-Hunter

Living With Periodic Paralysis:
The Mystery Unraveled

To Sandy, I will never forget.

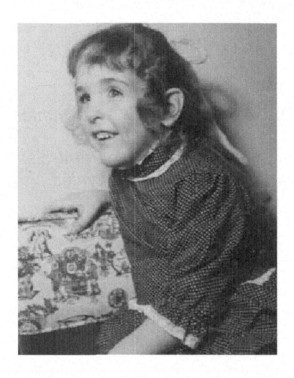

Contents

Foreword
Gerald I. Sugarman, M.D.,
F.A.A.P., F.A.A.F.P., J.D.

This is a wonderful tribute to a special memory of a special child – Sandy's " I Wanna Go Home" a study of Cerebral Gigantism – Sotos Syndrome. Written by her mother, Susan Knittle-Hunter, with the support of her husband, Calvin, both having degrees in special education and psychology, is a moving work on their life and times to Sandy's care. I am sure that many parents can relate to the daily activities necessary to care for these special children and how much of their days and nights are devoted to the care and needs of these children and in return, received their special love. A memory never to be forgotten, even though seemingly brief.

It is my privilege to write the foreword of this special book that will aid families, friends, health care persons, social workers, developmental specialists, nurses, clinics, pediatricians, orthopedists, family practitioners who share in the care, treatment and understanding of these loving children whether they have Sotos or related developmental syndromes. Sandy's story is well written, accurately detailed, and full of emotion and tragedy due to her untimely and unnecessary demise. It is reading for all to enjoy, reflect, appreciate, ponder, experience and learn. It was my pleasure having attended Sandy and her mother.

I first became interested in pediatric genetic syndromes early in medical school and internship at the Los Angeles County General Hospital in 1962 when I began cytogenetic chromosome karyotyping technique. I went on to become the director of the genetic clinic, the metabolic bone dysphasia clinic and the neurology clinic at Orthopedic Hospital in Los Angeles for 18 years. I have evaluated, treated and taught about syndromes for over 30 years. A lot has changed in the classification and nomenclature of syndrome, birth defects and genetics. I have published on Sotos syndrome associated with adult liver carcinoma (Am. J. of Children 131: 631-633 June 1977) and speculated at that time that this syndrome as well as other genetic syndrome control oncogene (genes that turn on the cancer cells). I went on to have four syndromes named after me because I published rare and interesting cases that were never published before.

Gerald I. Sugarman, M.D.

Dr. Gerald I. Sugarman diagnosed Sandy with Sotos syndrome in 1969 at Orthopedic Hospital in Los Angeles. Dr. Sugarman is a nationally known author and has published several books as well as more than 50 articles. He has a Master's Degree in Biochemistry from George Washington University and a M.D. degree from the Chicago Medical School. He is board certified, in both pediatrics and family practice. He is a Fellow of the American Academy of Family Physicians and a Fellow of the American Academy of Pediatrics. He has studied and published syndromes including Cockayne, the rare aging syndrome. He has been involved in the research of metabolic, neurological, and endocrine disorders for more than 30 years. Dr. Sugarman is also an attorney, having attended law school, receiving his J.D. in 1976. He specializes in medical malpractice cases for the injured child or adult.

Author's Preface 1 1993

I began writing this book fifteen years ago; five years after my daughter passed away. After outlining fourteen chapters and writing six chapters, I put the manuscript away while I raised my family and completed my education.

As a special education teacher and consultant, I see that many problems still exist for disabled children and their families today. Human rights are being violated daily. I felt it was time to complete this book and let the world know what a struggle it is to be the parents of a disabled child and how we, as a society, need to change the way in which services are provided to these families.

I have great respect and admiration for the families with whom I have worked over the years. They are truly the inspiration for completing this book.

Susan Q. K. Hunter, B.S., Salt Lake City, Utah July 1993

Author's Preface 2   2003

Since I completed writing Chapter One through Chapter Fourteen of this book in 1993, I have become disabled. My husband, Calvin, has assisted me in completing Chapters Fifteen through Chapter Eighteen and he is publishing the book in eBook format for me.

I had intended to go through the first thirteen chapters to change the words, such as "handicapped," to more updated and socially acceptable and approved forms ("challenged"). I also considered updating my knowledge of medical terms and Sandy's diagnosis. However, I have decided to leave the transcript as I originally wrote it. I feel the older terms and my lack of knowledge of medical terms and Sotos Syndrome, at the time the events unfolded, would aid the reader in understanding the impact of the events on me during my daughter's life and death.

This story takes place in the late 1960's and early 1970's. Many things have changed since that time in relation to the medical, educational and social aspects of having a child born with Sotos Syndrome. Today one has only to turn on a computer, type in the words "Sotos Syndrome" and all the knowledge is there that one needs to know about the syndrome. There are parents going through the same things just a click away. Education now exists for challenged children thanks to the passage of Federal Public Law 94-142; The Education for All Handicapped Children Act, which became law after Sandy, passed away. This law guarantees all children with disabilities the right to a free, appropriate and equal education. Social programs exist also, now, geared to assist families with all of the challenges that having a disabled child can bring. Some of the archaic training schools and institutions have been closed during the last 20 years.

Sotos Syndrome: A Tribute To Sandy

When Sandy was born and during her short five years of life, none of the above programs and opportunities existed. I felt very alone attempting to find any information regarding her condition and what to expect. I had to fight to get her an education. The social programs wanted me to "put her away" and "forget her" in one of those archaic institutions. I wish Sandy and I would have had the opportunities that families have today, when they discover their child has been born with Sotos Syndrome or any disabling condition.

Chapters Fifteen and Sixteen deal with my life and the changes I made after Sandy passed away and Chapter 18 includes an up-to-date overview about Sotos syndrome and the services available today for parents and children. We have attempted to write the information in "easy to understand" terms and format.

It has been nine years since I wrote the first preface in this book and nearly 30 years since Sandy passed away but, unfortunately, problems still exist in the educational, medical and social aspects of the lives of children and adults with challenges. It is my desire that this book will inspire and assist parents of children with Sotos Syndrome or any other challenging conditions, to fight for the rights of their children and themselves. I hope, also, that the teachers and professionals who work with these children; will fight for their student's rights and those of their student's parents.

Parents do not give up the fight!! Ask questions; read; study; learn all you can; push the doctors, teachers, school administrators, and professionals; learn; know and demand your rights and those of your child; demand to see specialists; and most of all, demand respect for you and your child!

Susan O. K. Hunter, B.S., Christmas Meadows, Utah 2003

Author's Preface 3   2003

Susan writes a powerful account of Sandy's daily life and death struggles. Susan's story clearly points out that children with disabilities are vulnerable, and adults need to take responsibility for their care and wellness. Anything less is unacceptable. Thank you to the people who cared about the sufferings of a helpless little child and her mother, and took the time and effort to offer help and comfort. You will never be forgotten. Susan and I have spent several decades working with children and adults with disabilities in a variety of public and private settings. Susan became totally disabled several years ago and was forced to discontinue work and doing the other things she really loved. It has been my privilege and honor to put Susan's and Sandy's heart felt story in print for the world to read. Sandy's life may have come to an early end but her memory will live forever.

Calvin Hunter, B.S., B.S., M.E.
Christmas Meadows, Utah May 29, 2003

Introduction 2013

It is the year 2013 and 40 years have now passed since Sandy's untimely and unnecessary death. Sadly, problems still exist in the educational, medical and social aspects of the lives of children and adults with challenges and health issues. This book and the story it relates is still relevant and could have been written today. Individuals are still dying from sepsis, negligence and malpractice in emergency rooms and hospitals around the world.

Organizations and groups are being created daily to fight these horrific injustices. Social networking has bonded people together who are victims or who have loved ones who are victims of malpractice and iatrogenic medicine. These organizations, networks websites and Facebook groups and pages advocate for change and offer support. They are bringing awareness to the suffering, maiming and death of innocent men, woman and children at the hands of those who are sworn to "do no harm."

I now belong to several advocacy groups and have my own advocate network. I am working towards medical safety in the ER and hospitals and better diagnosing of rare diseases. I have written another book about my own experiences with these issues. All of these many years later, things have not changed much, but there are more of us finding each other and working together to change the status quo of negligence and a lack of responsibility of the actions of doctors who are maiming and killing everyday.

I myself have been very ill for many years. I was misdiagnosed and mistreated with improper medications. Irreversible damage has been done and I am now permanently disabled in a power wheelchair hooked up to oxygen around the clock. I spend my days trying to make sure that this does not happen to anyone else ever again.

I have a daughter who died due to malpractice at the age of 5 and I have been maimed for the rest of my life. This has to stop. Sandy's message is still important today and this book needs to be republished as a second edition to spread the word that doctors who are negligent need to be held accountable and new methods for diagnosing patients correctly need to be researched and put into practice.

It has been 40 years since Sandy passed away. This Christmas will be her 46th birthday. She has missed 41 years of birthdays, holidays, life with her family, vacations, graduations, weddings, the birth of new family members, the passing of beloved family members, graduations, meeting new friends, moving to new places and the joy of being alive and being loved. I have missed sharing all of that with her. There is no way to make up for it. The pain is nearly unbearable when I think about it. No doctor was ever held accountable for taking my daughter away from me is such a cruel manner.

Sandy's life and death still must have meaning, even 45 years later. Nearly everyone is gone now who knew Sandy, loved her or who remember her, but it is my hope that anyone who reads this book will know her, and love her. I also hope the readers will find meaning in her story and in remembrance of her may join an organization or network and fight for changes in medical safety and patient advocacy.

.

This book was self-published in an eBook format in 2003 and reached many people. Technology and low costs today makes it possible to finally publish it as a paperback book. This is something I always hoped to do. This makes it possible to reach more people.

As in 2003, for the Second edition I have again decided to leave the transcript as I originally wrote it except for making a few technical changes and updating some information. Then as now, I feel the older terms and my lack of knowledge of medical terms and Sotos Syndrome, at the time the events unfolded, would aid the reader in understanding the impact of the events on me during my daughter's life and death.

Susan Q. Knittle-Hunter, B.S., B.S.
Sequim, Washington November 2013

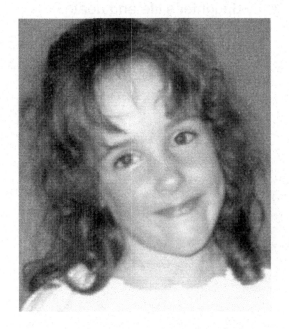

CHAPTER ONE

THE BEGINNING

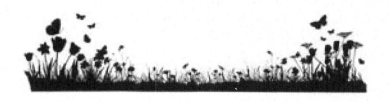

It is a blustery winter day in 1987. I am sitting in the living room of a middle class home in Salt Lake City, Utah. The room is filled with professional people. This intake meeting is being held to place a mentally disabled boy into a small group home.

I am a Program Coordinator and Consultant for the Division of Services to the Handicapped for the small group home program in Salt Lake County. This program involves moving the patients from the Utah State Training School for mentally disabled individuals into small group homes. These homes are much like foster homes. A regular family may have up to three disabled children placed with them. They are trained to provide the services necessary to the children and are also provided trainers (trained specialists) to go into the home daily to assist with the needs of the children.

The other professionals in attendance at this meeting include a social worker, an intake worker, the case manager, the professional parents and the group home trainers. One other important person is present; the boys natural mother. We are telling her about all of the wonderful services her son will receive, how well he will be taken care of and all of the assistance the group home parents will receive.

After listening quietly she finally begins to speak, obviously feeling overwhelmed. She is visibly shaken and begins to cry. When she regains her composer she angrily tells us her feelings. "I had to place my son at the Training School because I could get no help. I could not handle him and his problems by myself. It was the hardest thing I ever had to do. I have suffered extreme guilt and pain. I have cried myself to sleep many nights. And now, suddenly, I get a call telling me that my son is being moved from the Training School and being placed in the home of a family that I do not know. You are going to provide that family with anything and everything they will need to care for him." She sobbed, "Why can't you let me have him back and give me the help?"

She is right! What an injustice and I am part of it! I know exactly how she feels. I understand. I am the only person in this room who has true empathy for this mother.

I can feel a stinging in my eyes and pain in my stomach. I am shivering. I cannot speak. Many years before I had to give up my own disabled child when she was only two years old because I had no help, no one who really cared or understood. The memories flood in.

I remember back to 1966, shortly after my graduation from high school, in Venice, California, a suburb of Los Angeles. I met Bruce through an old friend. We liked each other immediately. He was in the army at the time; having just completed basic training. We saw each other on weekends and when he got leaves.

Bruce was a very pleasant young man and treated me very well, as well as my daughter, Tamara Marie (Tammy) born while I was still in high school the year before. He appeared to love Tammy and accept my situation. He was quite sensitive and easy to love. After four short months we decided to marry in April of 1967.

Chapter One: The Beginning

We thought we could be together because during basic training Bruce had been injured in an accident and was told that he would not be going to Vietnam with the rest of his battalion. We assumed that he would be stationed in the United States and Tammy and I could accompany him. Six weeks later, however, he got his orders for Vietnam and left right away.

Soon after he left I discovered I was pregnant. I was delighted but at the same time discouraged for I realized that I would not be able to work and must remain with my parents until Bruce returned.

The months that followed were very difficult both physically and emotionally. I was quite ill for most of the pregnancy. Emotionally, it was extremely trying. Here I was 19, and pregnant for the second time without a husband nearby to help. He was in Vietnam and every day I worried about his safety. To add to my problems, my mother was not fond of Bruce and she chose to let her feelings be known. There were many occasions during that period of time when she would say cruel things to me about my husband or my new baby. Because I was so ill, I felt trapped. I lived for the day when my husband would return and we could finally be a family.

One day when I was seven months a long I got my first indication that something could be wrong with my baby. I began having severe pains. No one was around at the time to help me, so I had to take a bus to the doctor who was ten miles away in the next town. My doctor informed me that I was in labor, but at only seven months my baby would not have much of a chance to survive. She gave me some kind of a shot in my back. The pain stopped and everything appeared to be normal for the time being.

Several weeks passed and Christmas Eve befell us. My parent invited my three brothers and their families over for dinner and to celebrate a day early. We all had a wonderful time and everyone spoke of the possibility of my having a Christmas baby. Of course I laughed, for I knew my baby was not due for another month.

I was really looking forward to this Christmas because it was the first year that Tammy understood what the holiday was all about. I could hardly wait for Christmas morning to see her face. It all helped ease the pain of Bruce being in Vietnam.

A few minutes before midnight my parents and I finally got to bed after playing Santa. At the stroke of midnight I had a terrible contraction that would not let up. My mother called the doctor and then took me immediately to the hospital. Little did I realize, as I felt my first labor pain, that my life was about to change more drastically than the normal ways of a new baby coming into a family and a way that would change the rest of my life.

I do not remember much of what happened after my arrival at the hospital. I slipped in and out of consciousness for the next twelve hours. My mother later told me that I nearly died. Due to complications, a specialist was called in and a caesarian section was almost necessary.

It was a very difficult delivery, but at 12:33 PM on Christmas afternoon, Sandra Renissa (Sandy) was born; weighing 7 lbs, 8 oz, and measuring 20 inches long. I got just a glimpse of her before I fell into unconsciousness again.

I awoke in my room with mixed emotions. I recall feeling quite alone and depressed. I longed to be with

8

my husband and daughter. I asked a nurse for some stationary so I could write my husband. She said it was impossible for me to sit up yet, so I would have to call him. When I explained that he was in Vietnam, she pardoned herself and quickly left the room. As I lay there I realized I had missed Christmas morning with all its excitement. To add insult to injury the nurse brought me a plate of cold cuts for dinner rather than the traditional turkey and trimmings. It was a good thing my parents had an early Christmas dinner for us.

Somehow in all at the depression, I had almost forgotten my sweet new baby. A surge of excitement came over me. What a wonderful Christmas!

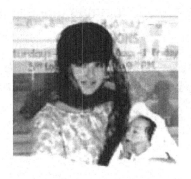

Baptism day.

CHAPTER TWO

FORT ORD

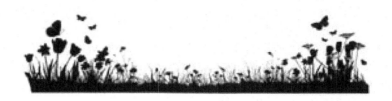

Not long after we had settled into our new home I decided that it might be a good idea to have a doctor at the base look at Sandy. It was about time for her six-month check-up and I was concerned about her leg. I talked to Bruce about it and he agreed with me.

I told him of the problems with Sandy right after he got home from Vietnam. He was resentful that I had not told him while he was overseas, but he did understand my reasoning. His reaction was to deny anything was wrong.

We made an appointment with a pediatrician. Bruce got a little time off to go with me. A nurse led us to a small room and instructed us to undress Sandy and lay her on the table. After a short while, a dark haired, middle-aged doctor walked into the room. He proceeded to look at our baby. He turned around and asked, "Is this all she does, just lay there?" We agreed affirmatively. He asked us to bring her back the next day. He wanted some other doctors to examine her. We were a bit puzzled by his request, but we agreed and set up another appointment.

It was all I could do to get through the rest of the day. Why did he want the other doctors to look at her? What was wrong with our baby? Bruce remained calm and refused to believe that there could be anything seriously wrong.

We returned as scheduled and we were very much surprised as a team of eight doctors marched in. They began to push and pull on her. They inspected every inch of her little body several times. Each one of them was making alarming comments to one another as if we were not standing there. Finally, after what seemed an eternity, an older doctor with gray hair appearing to be the head of the team looked around and said, "Your daughter has cerebral palsy."

My heart sank. I sat there in shock for a few moments. After I realized what it meant I began to cry. I did not know very much about the condition, but I knew enough to understand that our daughter could be seriously handicapped. Bruce did not say anything and appeared not to show any emotion.

After the initial shock, the doctor informed us that Sandy also had what appeared to be a deformed hip socket. All of the doctors agreed she should be hospitalized and placed in traction for several weeks, after which time they would operate to correct the defect or she may never walk.

We felt they must know what was best so we made arrangements to have her admitted to the base hospital the following morning.

As we were driving home Bruce asked me what the doctors meant by Cerebral Palsy. He had never heard of it before. As I told him the grim facts he again denied that our baby could be afflicted with anything so serious.

I find it difficult to describe the pain I felt as I watched my little baby being placed in traction the next morning. Her leg was pulled up in the air and taped to ropes that were attached to weights on the other end. Over the weeks they would increase the weight. She would have to lie there in the same position for at least six weeks.

My emotions were taken over with guilt. I began to wonder what I had done to cause this to happen to my sweet innocent baby. Had I done something so terrible that I was being punished in some way through my child? I could find no answer to ease my mind.

The weeks that followed were trying, to say the least. I did not like to see Sandy like that and yet I wanted to spend as much time with her as possible. We had only one car at the time so I had to wait for Bruce to get off duty every night to take me to the hospital. There was also the problem of who could watch Tammy for us during our visits. We had no family nearby. I remember crying myself to sleep every night worrying about our baby. This began to wear on our relationship. Bruce would not face reality and gave me little comfort.

As we were approaching the sixth week of Sandy's confinement we walked into her room one evening and noticed her foot was turning purple. We quickly called a nurse. She told us that she could not do anything for her without a doctor's order. We became quite angry and insistent. She put in a call to the doctor and said that he was due soon anyway. Bruce had to return to duty so we had to leave, but did so hesitatingly. We tried to believe that the doctors were professionals must know what they are doing.

The next morning we went to check on Sandy after several phone calls. We could hardly believe what we found. She was out of the traction, lying unconscious, with her foot and ankle bandaged. We had not been informed of any of this.

The doctor had not shown up and the traction had slipped until the tape had cut her foot to the ankle, all the way to the bone. The nurses did not help her until it was too late.

Now the surgery had to be postponed until her foot healed and then she would have to go through the traction all over again. The disappointment and anger were difficult to contain.

Two weeks passed and Sandy was still in the hospital recovering from the trauma. Bruce and I began to be more concerned. We had not seen her foot since the accident occurred. The doctors and nurses continued to put us off. They told us her foot was healing well.

We decided to go to the Chief of Staff. We told him that at this point in time we should be happy that her hip was healing, not her foot. We asked to have her released so that we could take her back to Los Angeles to have her treated there. We no longer were confident with what they were doing for our daughter. The doctor reluctantly agreed and discharged Sandy from their care. Bruce requested an emergency leave and we immediately headed for Los Angeles. Our first stop, after the long journey, was the emergency room of Orthopedic Hospital. My parents had phoned ahead for us, so they were expecting us.

We told them our story and they were very kind to Sandy and us. As they checked her foot they told us that we had done the correct thing. Sandy's foot was infected. They cleaned it and gave us some medication. They also showed us how to clean it. They let her leave with us. They felt there was no need to keep her in the hospital.

Chapter Two: Fort Ord

While examining Sandy, the doctor noticed what the other doctors had observed. He felt she might have Muscular Dystrophy. He suggested we bring her back in a week to have her foot looked at and some x-rays taken of her hip and be seen in the clinic again. Maybe they could come up with a conclusive diagnosis.

We left there quite confused. First we were told Sandy had Cerebral Palsy and now a doctor felt she could have Muscular Dystrophy. What were we to think?

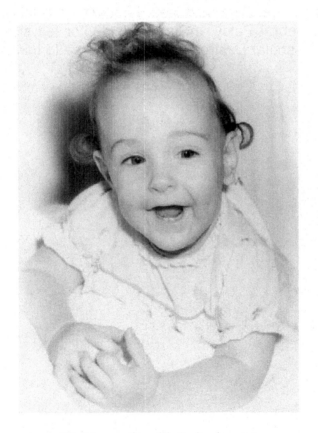

Eight months old. In body cast

CHAPTER THREE

BACK TO LOS ANGELES

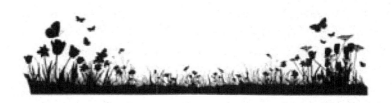

It was not an easy task to leave our new little dream house but after less than two months in Fort Ord, we decided to move back to Los Angeles. Proper medical attention for Sandy was our utmost concern. The children and I stayed with my parents until we were able to find an apartment. Bruce applied for a hardship discharge for an early dismissal from the army but had to stay behind at Fort Ord until he was officially discharged. By the end of July we were in our own apartment and Bruce had been reinstated to his previous civilian job, as a printer operator

On Sandy's next visit to the clinic at Orthopedic Hospital an orthopedic specialist examined her and took some x-rays. We were delighted to discover that surgery was not needed. The doctor felt that putting her into a body cast (spica cast) with her right leg in the appropriate position for six weeks should correct the hip problem. If it did not work surgery would then be indicated, but he was very optimistic about the outcome.

The doctor had us prepare Sandy for the cast by having us do special stretching exercises for her hip and leg and he prescribed her to wear a special splint called a Freijka pillow. The pillow was oblong, about an inch thick covered with canvas material and had straps attached to it. The straps fastened at the shoulder after it had been folded in half pulling her legs into a frog leg position. She had to wear it at all times except for diaper changing and bathing.

It took several weeks for Sandy's foot to heal completely. The unfortunate incident had left an ugly scar on her ankle one inch long and one-half inch wide. We were told that only plastic surgery or skin grafting would cover it up or remove it. We were quite angry to think that such a thing could happen in a military hospital. We considered suing the military but we were discouraged. We were told we could not sue the government. I am still filled with anger when I think about it today.

On July 19, 1968, at almost eight months of age, Sandy was placed in a bilateral frog leg spica cast. She was to remain in it for at least six weeks. The cast covered her body from her chest to her toes on her right side and just to her knee on her left side. Both legs were in a frog-like position. There was an opening in the diaper area for sanitary reasons. A diaper could easily be slipped in and a large pair of snapping plastic pants worn over it. Sandy never seemed bothered at having to wear the cumbersome frame although it appeared to be terribly uncomfortable. She always remained her sweet congenial self and was always ready with a smile.

Because of Sandy's size it was not too terribly difficult to take care of her or push her in a stroller, which I often did. We had a station wagon so it was not difficult to travel with her. She could lie in the back and with the aid of pillows, not slide at all.

As I looked upon my sweet little baby lying in the heavy, stiff cast, I often felt the same pangs of guilt I had felt seeing her lying in traction. During that same period of time something else began to bother me.

People's reaction to seeing Sandy in the cast was something I had never experienced.

I never realized how insensitive the general public could be. For some unknown reason, it was assumed that we had done something to our baby to cause her to be in the cast.

For instance, one weekend we decided to join the rest of our family on a camping outing in Sequoia National Park. The doctor told us it would be just fine as long as we kept her clean and dry.

One afternoon we were pushing Sandy along in her stroller at the village, when a woman came up and asked very angrily, "What did you do to your baby?" Bruce could not resist and quipped back, "We threw her down two flights of stairs!" Of course, the woman was upset, grunted something and stormed away.

I really did not mind if someone came up and seemed genuinely concerned. I would be polite and talk with them. Some people, however, did not deserve that consideration.

One particular incident comes to mind. My mother and I decided to go shopping one sunny afternoon. We, of course, took the children, pushing Sandy along in her stroller. We had just left a department store, had crossed the street and had walked about a block when a woman standing in front of the store began yelling for us to wait. We thought perhaps we had forgotten something. We waited for her and could hardly believe our ears when she ran up and asked, "What's wrong with your baby?" My mother and I looked at each other and then down at Sandy and then my mother replied, "I do not see anything wrong, do you Susie?" I replied,

"Not a thing." Then we turned around and continued walking.

We had a few problems arise while Sandy was in her cast. One night she developed a bad case of diarrhea. It was a terrible mess. We took her to the clinic the next morning fearing they would have to remove the cast and start all over again. As luck would have it, they were able to repair the damage with no real problem other than to add more weight to the cast.

One experience, which added to the terrible guilt I already carried, happened on a warm summer morning. I had to walk to the nearest post office to pick up an important letter. As Tammy and I walked along pushing Sandy in the stroller, we came to a long strip of sand in place of sidewalk (we were only a block from the beach). We had no choice but to attempt to get through it with the stroller. As I pushed, the front wheels got caught and Sandy slipped right out and fell face first into the sand. People stopped to look at poor little Sandy, not one of them offering to help and me. I will never forget the humiliation I felt. I cried and cried.

I only wish people would have tried to understand or put them into our situation. We were doing the best we could. People were always quick to criticize or give advice but no one really gave us credit for doing as well as we did. It was not easy for us to bear such a burden and no one knew the guilt that we carried. Nothing in our lives to that point had prepared us for what we were dealing with.

The six long weeks passed. We were very excited as we arrived at the clinic that morning. Our excitement turned to frustration as the doctor informed us that Sandy had to remain in the cast for another four weeks. I became terribly upset. I did not think any of us could stand another month, but the doctor reminded me of how important it was for her hip to heal completely. She might have to have surgery or she may never walk if we did not take every precaution. I knew he was right, but he did not have to live like we did. Begrudgingly, we left for another month of the same problems.

Thinking back, it was not Sandy who minded the cast. She always remained cheerful, letting little bother her. She was easily occupied and kept herself entertained. Our television became her electronic babysitter.

Four more long weeks passed and the big day finally came. The cast was finally removed, but what a terrible experience it was. What we thought would be a happy event turned into a nightmare. The doctor used some kind of an electric saw that made an awful noise. It was very frightening for Sandy. She screamed through the entire experience. It was worse for her than the entire ten weeks she spent in the cast. We have often discussed since that time the real necessity of using such a saw on a young child.

When the cast was finally removed we could see that Sandy's legs were shriveled and stiff. We were told of the importance of being careful with her. The cast had been sawed in half and the lower half was preserved because she was to remain in it most of the time. She could only be taken out for two hours a day. After a few days we were again to place her in the Freijka splint for most of the time.

We were elated as we left the clinic that day. Sandy was finally out of the cast. It would not be long now before she would be able to crawl and then walk like other children, or would she? The cast, with all of its problems, had diverted us from the unsettled questions. Now we could have all of the tests

21

preformed that the doctors and we were anxious to have done. Maybe we could finally know what was wrong with Sandy.

CHAPTER FOUR

SANDY LEARNS TO CRAWL, STAND AND WALK

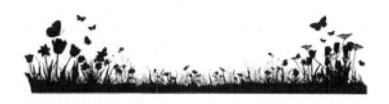

Hardly a week had gone by from the day that Sandy had her cast removed when she suffered a setback. For a little while each day we would sit her on the sofa propped up with pillows so she could strengthen her muscles and learn to sit by herself. One afternoon the pillow slipped and she fell forward. As she did, we heard a loud popping noise and then she started to cry as if in a great deal of pain. Her leg began to swell so we rushed her to the hospital. They took some x-rays, but luckily everything was all right. I was so afraid that she would have to be put back in the cast.

By Sandy's first birthday she was still not sitting by herself. We began to be concerned and of course we remembered the different opinions and diagnoses. Some tests had been completed but nothing conclusive had resulted. She was finally scheduled to see two neurological pediatricians; Dr. Smith and Dr. Sugarman.

Dr. Sugarman examined Sandy and decided to put her in the hospital for five days of testing including a muscle biopsy because of the delay in her motor development. There was a possibility of muscle involvement. It was to be a minor operation in which a piece of muscle tissue was removed from her leg and studied.

Sotos Syndrome: A Tribute To Sandy

On January 30, 1969 Sandy was admitted to the Orthopedic Hospital in Los Angeles. The following day the procedure was performed by Dr. Smith, taking approximately one hour. Muscle tissue was removed from her left leg. It was almost more than I could bear seeing my sweet baby unconscious and being wheeled into, surgery. It was only a minor thing but, never the less, frightening for us all.

She came out of the surgery well, but now she carried three scars for the first year of life.

During the five days other tests were run including an electromyogram, an electroencephlogram and a chromosome count. I was able to be with Sandy for most of the five days so it was not as frightening for her. I was able to feed her and be with her for most of the testing. I don't remember that anyone else other than Bruce came to the hospital to visit her.

She was released on the fifth day. We were not told any of the test results at that time. It was several weeks before we were called in to confer with Dr Smith. At that time Bruce could not leave work so my father took me in for the appointment.

I do not like to think about that day. It was probably one of the most difficult of my life the doctor asked me to leave the examining room while he observed Sandy. I remember that time seemed like an eternity. Finally, a nurse asked me to meet with the doctor in his office. I was not prepared for what he had to tell me. In a cold, matter of-fact manner he told me that my daughter was mentally retarded. His conclusion came from the previous testing and his own observations and findings. He did not know the degree of retardation; we would not know for a few years.

24

Chapter Four: Sandy Learns To Crawl, Stand And Walk

I remember being stunned. The words hit me like a knife going through my heart. I tried not to cry but it was impossible to fight back the tears. I knew the most difficult thing was going to be telling Bruce. How would he take it? He had already refused to believe that anything was seriously wrong.

I made the terrible mistake of telling him over the phone while he was at work. He became very upset and began to cry. He hung up the phone and left work for the rest of the day. I did not see him until late that night. Things were never the same between us after that day.

Not long after that I conferred with Dr. Sugarman. He agreed with the Doctor Smith's opinion. Sandy was mentally retarded. His conclusions from the testing, previous records and his own observations led him to diagnose her retardation as a symptom of a very rare neurological disorder called Cerebral Gigantism, also know as Sotos syndrome. Her growth rate had been double since birth and all of her symptoms brought him to that conclusion. Children with this disorder are of the large brain syndrome, so their growth rate is extremely fast, they have some degree of retardation, elongated faces, flushed cheeks and usually poor coordination. It was such a rare condition that little research had been done on it at that time. There were no answers for us as to how or why it happened.

I remember the doctor jokingly telling me that I was lucky to have a girl because he had seen one boy with Sotos syndrome who was only six years old and weighed 100 pounds and had the height to go with it! He chuckled that she would be a "bruiser" and I should put her to work in the kitchen!

Dr. Sugarman was pleasant, easy-going and had a sense of humor. He made all of this easier to understand and cope with. He was always straightforward and to the point. He was also one of the few doctors that I felt I could really believe. If he did not know something he would admit it. It was refreshing to deal with a doctor who didn't treat us as if he were some all-knowing god!

As time progressed we grew to better accept the information we had received. Things were never easy but we now knew, more or less, what to expect. It would take Sandy longer to learn things like crawling, walking and talking; if she would do them at all. It also meant that we, as her parents, would need a great deal of patience, love and understanding if we were to help her grow and obtain her full potential.

We were to continue to take Sandy to Orthopedic Hospital to the different clinics every couple of weeks. There were the orthopedic clinics, pediatrics, neurological pediatrics, physical therapy, x-ray, laboratory and the brace shop for splints and special shoes. It seemed to never end. Of course the medical bills were tremendous and Bruce didn't make very good money at the time. We were lucky to qualify for Crippled Children's Services, which paid for most of what our insurance did not cover.

Between the routine visits Sandy would have to be taken to the pediatric clinic for high fevers, respiratory problems and allergic symptoms. Very few weeks would go by without some sort of problem. After awhile we took it in stride; it became a part of our lives. The guilt never left me and I never stopped worrying about her. It was never easy.

26

Chapter Four: Sandy Learns To Crawl, Stand And Walk

My marriage suffered greatly. Bruce had a difficult time accepting all of the problems. He never really did accept the fact that she was mentally retarded. I felt he blamed me in some way for everything. My own mother could never accept Sandy as she was. She once told me she resented her for being born the way she was. She never wanted much to do with her. She would avoid her whenever possible or do nice things for Tammy but not for Sandy. Some other family members had a difficult time dealing with her retardation.

Bruce's father told me one day that I must have done something to cause it. His mother lived back east and never saw her but she made it clear in a letter that whatever was wrong with Sandy did not come from her side of the family! We did get quite a bit of support from my father. He was always there when I needed help. He loved Sandy and felt that she was really special.

As time went on Sandy began sitting by herself. She later developed a technique of getting around by rolling. It was quite curious to see. We would laugh as we watched her, thinking it was cute but we still wondered if she would ever crawl.

We took her to the physical therapist and she suggested we make her something like a skateboard which we could strap her to and then help her to move her arms and legs. It took much work and a great deal of patience but within several weeks we finally had her crawling.

One afternoon I was almost sorry she had learned to crawl. It was around 4:30 in the afternoon and the girls were watching television in the living room. I was in the kitchen preparing dinner. I suddenly heard car horns honking in front of our apartment. (We lived on a very busy boulevard in an apartment complex, the third apartment back.) Something told me to find out what was going on. As I walked into the living room my heart sank! Our screen door was open and Sandy was gone! I ran out of the door in a panic and could hardly believe my eyes. Someone had left the front gate open and Sandy had crawled all the way out to the boulevard and crawled passed the cars onto the center divider and was sitting there with smile on her face as all the cars honked at her. Not one person got out of their car to move her or help her. Of course I ran out there in a panic and snatched her up into my arms.

I laugh when I think about that incident today, although, it was not funny at the time.

More time passed and Sandy began to pull herself up to stand, but she could only stand for a few seconds at a time. The physical therapist suggested a standing box. My father looked at one and then made one for her. It was built with just enough room in it for her to stand; she could not sit down in it. It was as high as her chest leaving her arms and hands free. My father put a tray on it so she could play or eat as she stood. We were to leave her in it for several hours a day to get her used to standing and to strengthen her legs.

At the age of twenty months Sandy finally began to walk unaided, a feat we were never sure would happen! The more she stood and walked, however, it became more evident that there was a problem with her feet and legs. Her legs were very bowed and she walked on the inside of her feet (almost her ankles).

She was quite a sight to see but it was beautiful to us just to see her finally walk!

CHAPTER FIVE

OPERATION AND CASTS

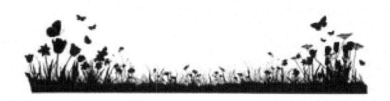

Due to the problems and pressures involved with Sandy's care, Bruce found it difficult to cope so we separated. During that time I took a trip with my parents to Pennsylvania to visit   relatives. I took Tammy and Sandy. We had a wonderful and relaxing time. We were gone for nearly a month.

When we returned Sandy's problems were more and more evident, but Bruce decided to make another go of it with the kids and I. We were so young to have these kinds of problems! It just did not seem fair.

Not long after returning from the trip Sandy was scheduled for her bi-annual visit to the orthopedic clinic. Upon examining her, the doctor decided that she should have surgery to straighten her legs and feet. He wanted to do a Grice Procedure. It is usually performed on children born with clubfeet. Sandy's condition was called calcaneovalgus deformity; mild rocker bottom feet (a turning of the heel bones). The procedure involves taking bone from the lower leg and grafting it into the foot to hold the bones in the correct position.

And so, once again, arrangements were made and at two years and one month of age Sandy was back in the hospital.

This time the operation was of a more serious nature and she was under anesthesia for a longer period of time. Of course there was recovery time, recuperation and rehabilitation periods to deal with.

All of these things were overwhelming. But the worst part was sitting in the hospital waiting and worrying about how she would come out of it.

It was difficult to deal with things and try to cope with Bruce's reaction to everything which was usually immature with a bit of denial.

It took several hours to complete the operation because the doctors had to place her lower legs and feet in casts. They were necessary to make sure the bones fused together correctly.

As she was wheeled passed us out of surgery my heart broke once again. My poor little sweetheart was going through more pain. Was it my fault? The guilt was unbearable. Bruce and I cried in each other's arms.

She had to stay in the hospital for several days. I was thankful that the hospital staff allowed me to stay all day with her. I did not like having to leave her at night. I knew it was all so frightening for her. Bruce would drive me the 30 miles each morning before he went to work and then pick me up after he got off of work.

The days seemed like an eternity, but we were finally able to take her home. We had six weeks to look forward to with her new casts. She was not able to put any weight on them or stand for fear the bones would not heal correctly.

The first several days were very trying. She was too heavy to carry so I was unable to go grocery shopping, etc. We decided to rent a wheel chair, which made things much easier for us. I remember once, however, trying to grocery shop by myself with the children. I tried pushing the wheelchair and the grocery cart and keep track of Tammy at the same time. It was a nightmare. After that, I took someone with me to help or I left the kids with a sitter.

Towards the end of the six weeks Sandy became restless. She wanted to stand and walk. It was a struggle keeping her down but it was wonderful thinking of her walking with nice straight feet and legs.

The happy day finally arrived and the casts were removed. They were carefully sawed down the middle of each side so that we could use the bottom sections to strap her into several hours each day. With the casts off we saw that once again her legs had shriveled and we saw three more scars, one on her lower leg about two inches long and one on each foot near her ankle about one and one-half inches, but her feet and legs were now straight.

The next test would be to see if she could stand on them. That took awhile because she had to gradually rebuild her muscles. It was not long before she was finally up and around. What a wonderful sight it was to see her walking and running on strong, straight legs and feet! It had all been worth the pain and problems involved.

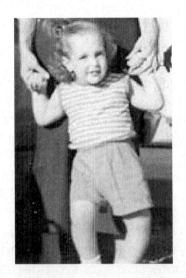

Finally standing. Bowed legs.

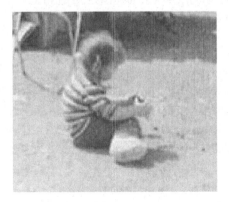

At family picnic. In casts after surgery.

CHAPTER SIX

A NEW BABY

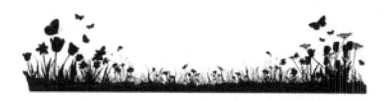

With things tending to normalize in our life, I began to think of things other than casts, hospitals, etc. I began to ponder things that had been shoved aside for a while.

Bruce and I had married in Las Vegas by a Justice of the Peace. With my Catholic upbringing I could never be happy with that. I contemplated a Church wedding by a priest. Bruce was not Catholic but agreed, knowing what it meant to me.

We had some counseling by a priest who told us we would have to stop using birth control. I disagreed with him because of the problems with Sandy. We did not need another child at this time. He said it was the only way he would marry us in the Church.

I had seen a marriage counselor during the time that Bruce and I had separated. He believed that having another child that was normal would help stabilize our rocky relationship. Putting both ideas together, Bruce and I decided to stop using birth control. I became pregnant almost immediately.

Unfortunately, Bruce reacted very negatively. He refused to marry me in the Church and decided to leave me. And so, for the third time, I was pregnant and alone.

Sotos Syndrome: A Tribute To Sandy

I was extremely confused, depressed and physically ill. I had no means of transportation. I had to go on welfare and had to rely on my parents once again for all my needs.

On our next visit to Orthopedic Hospital for Sandy's check up following the removal of her cast, I met with the social worker that had been following our case. I told her of my new situation. Sandy had become extremely aggressive and at times had terrible tantrums. She was too much for me to handle both physically and emotionally.

It was advised by the doctors and social workers that I place her in an in-patient setting until the new baby was born. I did not want to do it. I wanted to keep my 'baby' with me but I could no longer handle the situation alone.

The arrangements were made to place her in a home for handicapped children. The facility chosen was Angel View in Desert Hot Springs, 150 miles south of Los Angeles in the desert.

Several weeks passed as I made the preparations. I continued to hope that something would happen to change the plans. However, Bruce disappeared, my mother wanted Sandy to go and all of the professionals continued to press me in that direction. There was no one to turn to and I could find no other way out at the time.

CHAPTER SEVEN

SANDY GOES AWAY

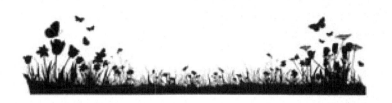

The fateful morning arrived. Sandy's clothes and toys were packed. Her name had been placed on each article carefully with love. Sweet little Sandy did not understand what was about to happen to her. Her comfortable little world was about to change drastically.

The social worker arrived very early since it was such a long drive. Tammy went with us. We drove for several hours making small talk and not talking very much about what was to happen. I just could not bear it.

We arrived shortly before lunchtime. Angel View was a modern looking, single-story and brick building on a hill overlooking the desert. We walked passed a swimming pool and I was told that part of Sandy's therapy would include swimming. We walked in the door to a very clean and hospital-like environment. Everyone was extremely friendly. I was asked to sign the guest book at the front desk. We were given a tour and we met about thirty other children. They were each handicapped in some way. We were invited to have lunch with the children. Everyone sat around several tables put together as one. Nurses and aids fed the children who could not feed themselves.

I could hardly swallow a bite. Tears welled in my eyes. I just wanted to grab my girls and run. Finally it happened. The social worker announced it was time for us to leave. I hugged and kissed Sandy and told her I loved her while tears streamed down my face. Sandy looked at me with puzzled eyes. She did not understand. As we walked down the hall toward the door I could hear her crying. She did not want me to leave her.

I did not say a word all the way home. I cried most of the time. I wanted my baby but I could not see her for six, long weeks. It was the rule at Angel View in order to let the child adjust.

Things seemed so quiet and lonely after we arrived home. Tammy and I missed her so much.

The next weeks were very difficult. I cried myself to sleep every night. I called Angel View to see how Sandy was doing as often as I could afford to, each time barely able to speak due to holding back my tears. The weeks seemed like an eternity. I felt so guilty leaving my child so far away with her not being able to understand why.

I tried to keep myself busy by visiting with my family and entertaining Tammy. She loved all of the attention that was now hers alone.

Six weeks had finally passed and I could now visit with Sandy. My parents offered to drive Tammy and me to Desert Hot Springs to see her. We planned to take her on a picnic in a near-by park. I was so excited.

We pulled into the parking lot. It was summertime and so very hot in the desert. As we walked through the front door the air conditioning was a welcome relief. We approached the front desk and signed the guest book.

A nurse or aid went to find Sandy. We watched her as she went down the long corridor. A few minutes later we could see her coming back with Sandy. Sandy started running with her funny little gait. She was squealing, "Mommy, Mommy." I was thrilled, but as she reached me she put her hand up to my face and slapped me. I was devastated. I was already filled with such guilt. I knew she did not understand why I had left her and she definitely had a right to be angry.

I hugged her and cried, and that was all she needed to know that I had not forgotten her and still loved her. Then everyone else had a chance to hug and kiss her.

Not long after our reunion we were on our way to the park. We ended up having to go all the way to Palm Springs, another one half-hour drive, to find a park. We found a lovely one and spent a wonderful afternoon eating, playing and visiting. It was extremely hot, but we didn't notice it much in view of our circumstances.

Taking her back was very difficult. She did not want to go and I did not want to leave her. It was such agony to have to drive away.

My parents drove us out, every other Sunday. It was too far to attempt every week. Each visit we would sign the guest book. After a few visits we realized we were the only ones to sign the book for weeks at a time. Some of those sweet children never got a visit from their parents.

We went to the same park and enjoyed our time together even though the summer temperatures in the park were in the hundreds. After each visit I would get very depressed.

Weeks turned into months. Summer turned to autumn. Time was drawing near for the birth of my third child. The doctors and social workers suggested that I leave

Sandy where she was and plan on never bringing her home. They suggested that mentally retarded children cause too much trouble and require too much time. My new baby would be healthy and I should devote my time and energy to the new child and Tammy.

I did not agree with them and experienced more anxiety in trying to decide what plans to make. I decided to see the priest in another parish. I would walk two miles each way to counsel with him twice a week. He understood that I loved Sandy and I was her mother. She loved me and needed me. I could not forget her and allow this new child to take her place. She had feelings and concerns like other human beings.

On November 10, Jeffrey Andrew was born. He weighed 9 lbs. and 6 oz. and was definitely a healthy baby, which was quite a relief.

About a week before Jeff was born, Bruce showed up. He announced to me, "If the baby is a normal boy I will come back, if it is a girl I won't come back and if anything is wrong with it like Sandy, you will never see me again." Those words still ring in my head after all of these years, however, for reasons I do not understand, I accepted him back when he discovered that Jeff was a healthy baby boy and he asked me to take him back.

It turned out to be one of the bigger mistakes in my life. He would not allow me to bring Sandy home. He would drive us out to visit her. In fact, for Christmas and her third birthday she came home for a week, but he could not wait to take her back. I, on the other hand, loved having her at home with us.

Visits became further apart. He was trying to forget about her. I was so frustrated. I still had no transportation of my own and my parents refused to help me because I had gone back with Bruce.

The conflicts continued and we again separated. Bruce moved back to West Virginia. This time I filed for divorce and got a job. I did not want to go back on welfare, it was too degrading and demoralizing.

I had done PBX work previously and found an excellent job working as a receptionist for a prestigious bank in Century City. We moved into a small house in a nice neighborhood. A neighbor two doors away babysat for me. Everything was working out very nicely except for one thing. Sandy was still not home with us. I was now alone and did not know how I could care for the three children by myself, especially with Sandy's special problems. Was Sandy ever going to come home?

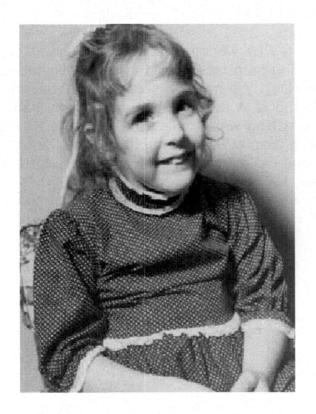

Christmas. Three years old.

CHAPTER EIGHT

ANOTHER PLACEMENT

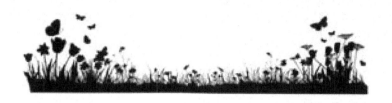

Over a year had passed since Sandy had been placed in Angel View. One day the social worker called me at work and told me that the director of the home wanted Sandy to be transferred. Angel View was a home for physically handicapped children. Sandy was totally rehabilitated physically: they had done everything they could for her. They felt she should now be placed in a home for mentally retarded children. Once again I was devastated. What was I going to do?

To put my mind at ease, however, the social worker related to me that tests had been preformed on Sandy and they had found the 'perfect' placement for her according to the results.

I managed a day off from work and the social worker took me to see the facility. I was appalled as we toured the facilities. It was a new home being filled with the most severely handicapped people from a nearby institution. There were adults mixed with children. There were auditorium-like rooms filled with crippled bodies lying on the cold floor. I saw only two children in the entire place who were ambulatory (could walk). As I walked around I felt myself detaching from my body. I was aware that people were speaking to me but I did not know what they were saying. I was in shock!

I could not allow these so-called professionals, who had supposedly performed testing on Sandy, to place her in that setting. This was all a mistake. She did not belong there. She could walk and run and play. She could talk and she could laugh. She would only regress. What was I to do? Who was going to help Sandy and me?

CHAPTER NINE

SANDY COMES HOME

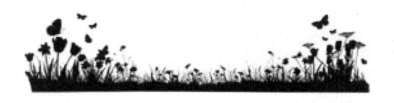

After much contemplation, in August of 1971, I decided that my only choice was to bring Sandy home. I knew that somehow I could make it.

The social worker's plan was to bring Sandy home on a Friday and allow her to visit with us for the weekend and then place her in the new home the following Monday. I went through the motions with her. I was afraid that I might not see Sandy again if I didn't. The children and I went with her on the long journey for the last time.

I was so relieved after I got Sandy in the car with all of her belongings. It was so exciting looking forward to a life with my three children together, at last!

Once I got home I proceeded to tell the social worker that I had changed my mind. I told her I disagreed with the results of their testing if, in fact, any had been done. I was going to keep Sandy home and proceed to have testing done on my own and find a placement for her, if that was necessary. I also made several phone calls to the other professionals involved and told them of my dissatisfaction and my new plans.

I felt quite proud of myself for being assertive and taking control of my own life and that of my children. I made an appointment with a leading pediatric neurologist at Children's Hospital in Los Angeles for a complete evaluation. The date for the examination was September 13, 1971, Veteran's Day, a local bank holiday. I would not have to miss another day of work.

The next several weeks were happy. Everything was working out very well. My neighbor agreed to sit for all three of the children. Everyone was adjusting. Sandy did not seem to have the aggressive tendencies she had displayed previously. Her temper tantrums had diminished almost entirely. She seemed happy to be home and we were happy to have her home.

Maybe things were finally going to work out for my children and me.

CHAPTER TEN

THE ACCIDENT

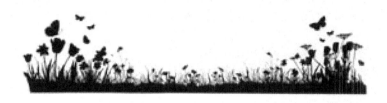

The morning of September 13 arrived. I was rather excited. The previous week I had purchased a compact, hatchback car from my brother and his wife. I was going to make monthly payments. I was finally independent and I was handling things well.

As I left that morning, I decided to leave Jeffrey with the babysitter. I was not sure how long the testing would last and thought it would be easier if I did not have to worry about him. Tammy, being older, was no problem.

The three of us got into the car. We drove a little while along the route my father had mapped out for me. I stopped for gas and noticed the time. It was getting late. I asked the attendant for the quickest way to Children's Hospital without taking the freeway (I had never driven the freeway before). He said that in order to get there at my scheduled time, I would have to drive the freeway.

Reluctantly, I found the freeway entrance and began driving. Everything was going along perfectly. Tammy sat next to me and Sandy had fallen asleep across the backseat.

Suddenly, a groove or lip in the road running parallel with the lane divider caught my left front wheel. Somehow, I lost control. We never found out exactly what caused the accident. The car rolled over toward the right on its side. We flipped four times. Each time just before we hit, I heard myself say; "Now I'm going to know what it feels like to be dead." It felt like an eternity before we stopped. We landed upside down.

I screamed for Tammy and Sandy. Tammy cried and answered but Sandy did not. I panicked. It was like some horrible nightmare. The only way out was through the window on the driver's side, the door would not open. I crawled out and then pulled Tammy out. She seemed to be all right except for a few cuts on her arm.

A man who had seen it happen ran over and showed me where Sandy was. She had been thrown out of the back of the car on the first impact. She was lying on the side of the road several hundred feet away. Many people were around trying to help her. I ran to her and thought for sure she was dead when I reached her.

Her eyes were filled with gravel, her left leg was in a circle; her right arm was thrown completely back and underneath her. I knelt down beside her and called her name. Then, miraculously, she said, "Mommy," softly. I talked reassuringly to her as a kind man covered her with a blanket and then informed me that a woman with a phone in her car had already called for an ambulance.

We had to wait for about ten or fifteen minutes for the ambulance. The freeway traffic had come to a total standstill. People were stopping to see what had happened and prevented the ambulance from getting through. I was so afraid Sandy would die before we could get her to the hospital. In my state of shock and hysteria I began yelling at the people to get moving. Some of the men helping Sandy tried to calm me down.

Chapter Ten: The Accident

Once the ambulance arrived, the paramedics worked quickly to get Sandy on a stretcher and into the vehicle. I asked them to take us to Orthopedic Hospital since the doctors knew us there and we were luckily not far away.

All the way to the hospital I continued to talk to Sandy attempting to keep her alive and reassuring her and Tammy that everything would be all right. I kept telling Sandy to "hang on." Tammy continued to ask me if Sandy was dead.

Upon arriving at the hospital, both girls were rushed into the emergency room. I never felt so alone and more afraid in my entire life. I called my mother and asked her to inform the rest of the family. She told me that they would all be there right away.

A policeman came and interviewed me for the accident report. He told me the car had been towed away and where I could find it. Luckily, I had not run into anyone and had not damaged any property. He told me it was a miracle considering the time of day and the heavy traffic that had developed. I was not cited, as there had been several witnesses to report that I had not been driving recklessly.

It was about an hour before I was told anything about the girls. For a while, they led me to believe that Tammy had also sustained some serious injuries. Finally, Tammy was released to me with a bandaged arm. Pieces of broken glass had lacerated her elbow, and other than being frightened, she was fine.

Sandy's condition was definitely more serious. At that point the doctors told me that they had cleaned the gravel out of her eyes, but she had a broken right arm and shoulder and broken left leg. She also had a large area on her upper left leg that had been lacerated. There was some type of internal injury because she was bleeding internally. Emergency surgery was indicated at that time, I signed a release form and she was immediately taken into surgery.

I was then examined and it was discovered that I had sustained a broken nose, a concussion and was very definitely in shock. I decided to see my own physician at a later date, after I knew more about Sandy.

During the surgery, which lasted several hours, Sandy's spleen had to be removed. It had been broken in half by the impact. It was explained to me that she could live without a spleen (an organ that fights infection in the body). The other organs in her body would take over its function. Since birth she had a poor immune system, so I was very concerned.

My parents finally arrived. It was comforting to have them near. Other friends and family dropped by throughout the evening.

After the surgery, a doctor informed me that Sandy was near death. They did not expect her to make it. They allowed my parents and me to see her. I almost fainted as I walked into the intensive care unit. She was lying naked and unconscious on the bed with a small sheet draped over her. She was hooked up to several machines monitoring her vital signs. Her legs and arms were straightened but not in casts. Her entire body was shivering and she was having difficulty breathing.

Due to how close to death she was, all of my brothers and their families were allowed a short visit with her. The doctors arranged for me to stay at the hospital that night for the same reason.

Chapter Ten: The Accident

My parents took Tammy with them and made arrangements for Jeff to stay with the babysitter. I did not sleep at all that night. I was so afraid and filled with such guilt over the accident. How could such a terrible thing have happened and why to Sandy? Had she not already been through enough in her short three years of life?

The next morning I met with the doctors again. Sandy had made it through the night! They felt she had been born a fighter and that was the only thing that kept her hanging on now. They insisted that I go home and take care of myself. They promised to keep me posted.

I took care of the necessary tasks at home and returned to the hospital. Sandy remained about the same. I returned home that night.

The following morning the phone rang very early and immediately, when I heard the doctor's voice, I knew something was terribly wrong. Sandy had sustained several broken ribs, which had in turn pierced her lungs. This had caused her lungs to collapse. They needed to do an emergency tracheostomy so she could breathe. I gave my verbal permission and rushed back to the hospital.

Hurrying into her room, I saw a strange metal tube protruding from her throat attached to a long plastic pipe, which was hooked up to a machine. The machine, a respirator, was breathing for her. Another incision had been made in her chest in which another tube was attached draining the fluid from her lungs. I wondered how much more her little body could take.

Shortly after that, I ended up in the hospital myself. I was still in shock and suffering from the concussion. I was scheduled to have my broken nose repaired.

Sotos Syndrome: A Tribute To Sandy

It was probably good for me to be resting in a hospital, but I worried the entire time about Sandy. I knew Tammy and Jeffrey were being well taken care of but Sandy still remained on the critical list. I remained in the hospital for two days and rested another day at home.

When I was finally able to see Sandy again she had been taken off of the critical list. I walked into her room and although she was still hooked up to the machines, she was now conscious. She recognized me and smiled. She could not talk, however, because of the tracheal tube in her throat.

It was wonderful to see some signs of improvement. The doctors felt that she had passed through the critical period and was now on the road to recovery.

Many of our friends and relatives visited her and brought her gifts. (Bruce was in West Virginia and never came to see her throughout the entire ordeal.) All of the love and attention helped to speed her recovery. She was taken off of the respirator and was able to talk and laugh again. She was quickly becoming her 'old self'.

Two weeks after the accident the doctors felt she was ready to go home. However, she again needed to be placed in a body cast for six weeks to two months due to her broken leg. That meant someone would have to take care of her full time at home.

I discussed it with my family and decided that because I could not afford a full time nurse, I would have to quit my job, go on welfare again and take care of her myself. It was going to be difficult but we could make it.

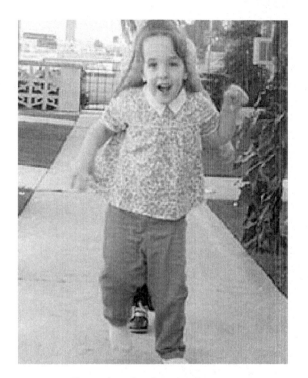

Running in the yard.

CHAPTER ELEVEN

SANDY COMES HOME AGAIN

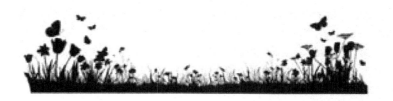

On September 19, sixteen days after the accident, Sandy came home from the hospital in a full body cast, from her chest to her toes. All of our neighbors and friends came to see Sandy and welcome her home. We were all so excited to be able to start over again. Hopefully, things would be better for us this time.

The cast had the familiar opening but this time we did not slip a diaper in it. Sandy was toilet trained so we were provided with a special slanted, wooden table on which she could lay on her back or her stomach. It had an opening for toileting. A pan was placed under the opening. We kept her covered across the middle section.

We placed her in the living room so she would not be alone and could easily be observed. The table had to be placed on the floor. The foot end touched the floor and the head end rose about a foot off of the floor. Sandy could play with her toys, look at books or color with her arms hanging over.

Taking care of Sandy this time was not as easy as when she was only eight months old. She was a very large girl for her age, due to her syndrome, and combined with the weight of a full body cast, it was impossible for me to lift her. It was all I could do to turn her every few hours. She could not be placed in a bathtub, so twice a day I gave her a sponge bath and every few days washed her hair in a bucket.

Since Sandy could not eat with the rest of the family, I ate every meal, with her on the floor. Sometimes Tammy and Jeffrey ate with us. It was difficult for her to feed herself in that position and with her lack of coordination, so I usually had to feed her.

The days became very long. Very few people came to see us, with the exception of my father, and it was unfeasible to go anywhere. It became quite lonely for the four of us. I was unable to grocery shop. I had to rely on my father for almost everything. It would have been impossible without his help.

One day, as Halloween was approaching, I began to worry about not being able to take Sandy trick or treating. I knew Tammy and Jeff were going to go with the neighbors but I wanted Sandy to have a fun time too. Then I had a wonderful idea. Why not bring Halloween to her! I talked to my father and together we planned a party for all of the neighborhood children.

On Halloween, after everyone went out to get their goodies, they all came back to our house. We played games, told scary stories and bobbed for apples. Sandy was involved in all of it and had a wonderful time. It was so good to see the kids having fun for a change.

The following week my father helped me take Sandy back to the hospital to have her cast removed. We were thankful for the help we received when we arrived. She was placed on a gurney and easily pushed from place to place.

Chapter Eleven: Sandy Comes Home Again

X-rays disclosed the bones were healed properly. The cast would for sure be removed. By now, Sandy was somewhat used to the saw and handled the procedure fairly well. The cast came off with little problem. However, until this time, the cast had covered most of Sandy's new scars. It was horrifying to see them. One scar went from her chest to below her belly button. There were several from the draining of the lungs and of course the large one across her neck from the tracheostomy. There was also a large, jagged, uneven scar about six inches long on her left thigh. It was not easy to hide my horror from Sandy. I attempted to be excited about the cast coming off, but inside I was riddled with guilt.

Although her legs were shriveled, we were told that Sandy could begin to stand and walk as much as she liked. We were also shown some exercises to help strengthen the muscles.

And so, without the cast, we left the hospital. For the first time in over two months Sandy was able to sit, stand and walk again. We were looking forward to a new life, once more.

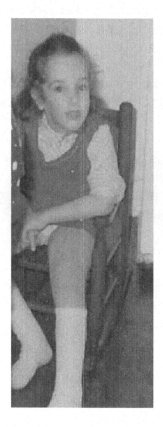

The day the body cast came off.

CHAPTER TWELVE

A NEW LIFE

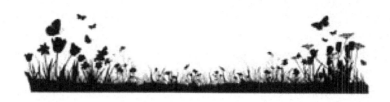

It took awhile for Sandy to regain strength in her legs, but not as long as I had anticipated. She was up and running in a matter of weeks.

However, one day, just when things were about back to normal, Sandy was playing on her big wheel in front of the house when she suddenly stopped breathing. Tammy ran to tell me. We rushed her to the hospital. For some reason her trachea had become blocked and she was unable to breathe. The doctors in the emergency room were able to save her, but she was admitted and placed in an oxygen tent for several days. She had developed pneumonia.

Within a week Sandy was home again, weak but happy. Was it ever going to end? How much more could we all take?

After the accident I had discovered a school for handicapped children existed just a few blocks from our home. I had read an article in the local paper about a Boy Scout Troop and a Girl Scout Troop for handicapped boys and girls sponsored through the school.

I took a chance and when Sandy was well enough I called and talked with the principal. She set an appointment for us for the following day.

The program was wonderful. It was a special school for handicapped children set up like a regular school. All of the children were handicapped in some way. Most of them were in wheel chairs or walked with braces and crutches. All of the children seemed happy and the teachers seemed well qualified and caring. The program was paid for by the Los Angeles Unified School District. Children, no matter what their problem, were provided an education for free. Every child was transported by school bus and attended school daily. They even provided a summer school program. Every child could live at home and still receive an education. (The interesting thing about this school was that it existed well before The Education of All Handicapped Children Act of 1975 [Public Law 94-142], which made it mandatory for all school districts to provide a free and appropriate education for all children no matter what handicapping condition existed.)

I did not know much about mental retardation but I was excited as I toured the school and learned about the things they had to offer and was sure that this was the appropriate place for Sandy. It was a dream-come-true! She could live at home with us and go to school every day. She could even receive speech therapy and physical therapy.

I was shocked, however, when the principal told me that Sandy was not "bad enough" to attend her school. I could hardly believe my ears. I begged and pleaded with her. I told her of our struggle and she finally agreed to accept her.

She began school the very next morning. The little, yellow school bus arrived on time and Sandy climbed aboard without hesitation. She smiled and waved as the bus pulled away. I could not contain my tears of joy knowing that everything was finally going to work out for us, especially Sandy. She was going to school like other children. She was laughing, walking and playing again. And now she was going to be learning like other children.

Now that Sandy had recovered and was in school, I felt I could go back to work. I hated being on welfare. I so much wanted to be independent.

I was lucky enough to quickly find a new job as a receptionist in a bank in Los Angeles. My father had to drive me every day in the beginning since I did not have a car and it was quite a distance from where we lived. I later transferred to a closer office and was able to purchase another car.

Things were going well for us. Sandy was able to stay fairly healthy and loved going to school. I had a good position, a car and was doing a nice job of raising my children on my own. I even began to date occasionally. Never before had I felt such satisfaction and dignity. For nearly a year, life was very pleasant. We had a few ups and downs, but for the most part things were finally stable. No one could have comprehended how our lives were about to change.

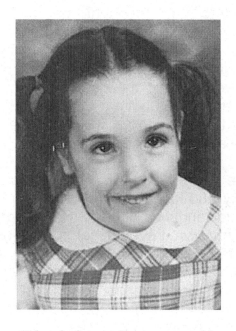

School picture. Four years old.

CHAPTER THIRTEEN

I WANNA GO HOME

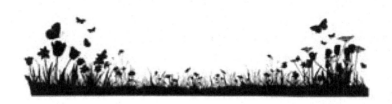

That Christmas, Sandy turned five. She had her first real birthday party on Christmas Eve. Some of her cousins and all of the neighborhood children arrived with gifts. She was thrilled and had a wonderful day with the children.

Christmas was very special for us too. We got together with the family for all of the festivities. Never had life been better.

During that holiday season a terrible flu was sweeping the country. Many people had actually died from it. I was unlucky enough to contract it a few days after Christmas. I was so ill that the children had to be farmed out to family and friends until I was well enough to care for them again. By New Years Day I was well enough to have the children home, but I was not totally recovered.

On January 3, the children were supposed to return to school. However, Tammy had a slight temperature and Sandy, although she did not have a fever, was not feeling well. Because the flu was so serious and Sandy had such a poor immune system, I decided to keep all of them home.

About an hour after I decided to keep the children home, Tammy called to me from the bedroom that something was wrong with Sandy. I ran in to find her face flushed, she was having trouble breathing and taking her temperature revealed a fever of 104 degrees. I immediately called our family pediatrician. (Dr. Morton had a practice in our neighborhood. She had agreed to see Sandy, with the knowledge of her problems, so we did not have to drive all the way into Los Angeles for the simple things.) Her only advice was to give her some aspirin and to tell me not to worry. I reminded her about Sandy's spleen having been removed making her more susceptible to infection. She treated me like I was overreacting and hung up.

Because I was still not feeling well, I called a neighbor to help me. Mary came right over and together we gave Sandy a cool bath and rubbed her down with alcohol. We took her temperature again and it had risen to 105 degrees.

I called the doctor again and this time she prescribed some medication. She also told me to bring Sandy into the office at 3:00 pm if she was not better by then. My father picked up the medication and we gave some to her right away.

After another few hours it was evident that the medicine, cool baths and alcohol rubs were not working. We were so shocked by her steady decline that we attempted to phone the doctor once again but she was out of her office. Sandy could no longer walk, she was saying that she could not hear and she was having problems with her vision. We decided to call the nearest emergency room.

The nurse that answered my call told me to give her a Popsicle and put her in another cool bath. I told her, "If Sandy could hold her head up and eat a Popsicle, I would not be calling." I told her that Sandy's condition appeared to be serious to us. She then conceded that we should bring her in to the hospital.

We left at 2:00 pm for the hospital. Mary drove us. We dropped Tammy and Jeff with my mother on our way.

When we arrived we were treated very rudely. The staff acted as if they did not want to be bothered with us. (I have always assumed that they believed I was overreacting). Mary had to leave and I was left alone to try and get help for Sandy.

First the doctor on-call examined her. He acted quite smugly. He did not believe that she had a temperature of 105 degrees. He asked Sandy questions about how she felt, etc. Since she spoke in only three or four word phrases and did not understand much of what he was saying, I explained that she was mentally retarded and I would have to answer his questions as well as I could for her. He got rude and said, "That's obvious." He then questioned me about all of her scars with disgust in his voice. I tried to explain the story quickly and made sure he understood about her spleen being missing. When he realized that her temperature was 105 degrees he quickly ordered a chest x-ray and some blood tests and then disappeared.

I was so afraid. I could see Sandy slipping away in front of my eyes and these professional people were treating us so poorly. I did not know what to do. No one was there to help me and I was exhausted. I was still sick myself and I had not eaten or rested all day.

After what seemed an eternity, a nurse and a lab technician walked in to draw some blood from Sandy. The technician made it clear to us that he did not want to be there. He had just returned from a vacation in

Hawaii and did not want to be back drawing blood. The nurse echoed his sentiment.

As the technician got close to Sandy to start the procedure, she began to cry and pull away. She had been through these things so many times that anyone dressed in white frightened her and she knew that whatever they were going to do would be painful.

I attempted to reassure and console her just as the nurse yelled at her to, "grow up," and proceeded to jump on her and hold her down with her weight while the lab technician got the blood. Sandy screamed in terror through the entire fracas. Then they hurried away leaving Sandy shaking with fear.

I could not understand this horrible treatment of both my sick daughter and myself. Sandy was extremely ill and needed medical attention, yet every medical professional we met treated us less than human.

Another nurse showed up a few minutes later, after I had calmed Sandy. She had come to take her to the x-ray department. Together we put Sandy in a wheelchair because she had deteriorated to the point that she could no longer stand or walk. She could no longer hold up her own weight in the chair. At that point, Sandy told me that she was afraid.

When we arrived at the department, the x-ray technician told me that Sandy had to stand up for the chest x-ray. I attempted to hold her up, but she kept slipping out of my arms due to her weakness. He took a picture anyway, but we were later told that it did not turn out. He relayed to me that we had to try another one. I had finally had enough and told him, "There is no way in hell this child can stand for the x-ray; you will have to find another way to do it."

He quipped, "I will make her stand, watch this." He found a roll of tape and a metal pole used for hanging IV's. He took Sandy's arms and pulled them above her head and taped her at the wrists to the pole. She was literally hanging off of the floor by her wrists. I started to argue with him about it when the doctor came in. He told us the first x-ray was good enough, and another one was not necessary.

The technician removed Sandy from the pole as the doctor explained that the x-ray showed her chest was clear and the blood work showed nothing to worry about, so he was sending us home.

Anger and frustration shot through me. I retaliated with, "You cannot send her home. She cannot walk or stand she is so weak. She is losing her vision and hearing. She has a fever of 105 degrees. You have to do something for her."

He explained that my family pediatrician had been informed of all the testing and was confident that Sandy needed only bed rest at home for recovery. Then a telephone was handed to me.

My pediatrician was on the other end. I tried to explain the situation. Her only reply was, "Take Sandy home. She only has the flu and has to suffer like everyone else." Then she hung up.

I was devastated. No one was going to help Sandy. No one would listen. No one cared. Was it because she was mentally retarded? Did she not have the worth of a normal child?

It was now 6:00 pm and I was in shock. I called my father and asked him to pick us up. He was unable to get there for two hours and no one else was available at the time to help.

During those two hours Sandy was allowed to sleep in a crib near the emergency room. A nurse came in once and complained that we were, "Using a bed that a 'sick' person could be using."

My father finally arrived at 8:00 pm. When he saw her condition he was quite surprised and questioned why we were taking her home. I told him how I felt about it, and explained what the professionals had told me. We reluctantly wheeled Sandy in a wheelchair to the car and took her home.

When we arrived at the house my father carried her in and on the way Sandy whispered in his ear, "Grandpa, you are my favorite one." He then had to leave right away.

I immediately put Sandy in another tepid tub. While I was holding her head up and pouring the water over her scar torn body, she looked up at me and said, "Mommy, I wanna go home." I said, "But Sandy, you are home now." She looked at me again and said wearily, "I'm not home yet." I somehow knew what she meant, but I did not want to believe it. I did not know how to help her any longer.

Just then my father returned with my mother and the other children. My parents had to work the following day so they could not take care of them for me overnight. They visited with Sandy for a few minutes and then left.

I got all three children ready for bed and then tucked each one into their blankets. As I got to Sandy I wondered if there was more that I could do for her. All of the professionals told me "Not to worry." "It's just the flu." "She had to suffer like everyone else." They had taken blood tests, and x-rays. They must be right. Maybe I just needed a good night of sleep, after all, I had been ill too. I could take better care of her tomorrow, if I got some rest. I kissed her and told her I loved her. Then I exhaustedly fell into bed, clothes and all.

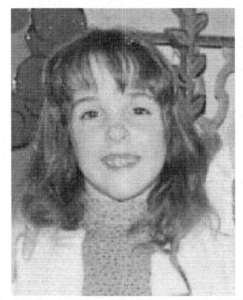

Last photo taken. New Years Eve 1973.

CHAPTER FOURTEEN

MY OWN SPECIAL ANGEL

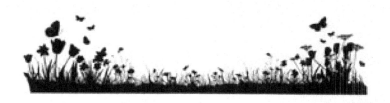

At 7:00 am I awoke with a start. I remembered Sandy. I ran to the girls' bedroom. I found her laying face down on top of her covers clutching her favorite stuffed animal. She was cold and stiff and her hands and feet were purple. She had obviously died, alone, soon after I fell asleep. She was apparently trying to get out of bed to get to me. I did not hear her.

Sandy had gone "home." Now my precious and sweet daughter was gone. My little girl; who cried every time she heard "Somewhere Over the Rainbow" in the Wizard of Oz, who loved to eat chocolate pudding, who loved to ride the school bus, who loved to listen to the Carpenters' and Simon and Garfunkle songs, who loved her "special grandpa", who loved to go for rides in the car, who loved to play with her cousins, who loved to go to school, who loved to get dressed up, who loved being with her big sister, who loved to watch cartoons on the television, who loved her baby brother, who loved to pick flowers, who loved to eat ice cream, who loved to ride her big wheel, who loved to sit on my lap, who loved everyone, was gone. She was gone. She was gone. My special little girl was gone. How was I going to say 'goodbye' to her? How could I put her in the cold ground? How could I leave her there?

I felt I had failed her again, or had I? No, no, no, it was the professionals: the doctors, the nurses, and the technicians! They had failed us! Sandy should have been allowed to stay at the hospital and the doctors and nurses should have attempted to save her life! They should have treated her with respect! They should have treated her as if they cared!

The next several days were a whirlwind of unbelievable feelings; pain, guilt, numbness, despair, emptiness, sorrow, anger, disgust, humiliation and degradation brought on by even more unbelievable occurrences.

I had to send her school bus away. The police came. Family members came. A hearse drove off with Sandy's body. The police made it a coroner's case. An autopsy was necessary because her pediatrician never came to the hospital to examine her, herself, so she could not sign the death certificate. Funeral arrangements had to be made. (A wonderful person, unknown to me still, paid for all of the arrangements since I had no insurance at the time.) A burial plot had to be chosen. The coroner fought with Dr. Sugarman for her brain. (The doctor requested it for research due to her unusual syndrome and the coroner just wanted it for his "collection.") I had to join the fight so Dr. Sugarman could have it for research. (I allowed this, hoping that the research may find a cause or cure for Sotos syndrome.) Her brain had to be divided, something that still sends shivers through me when I think about it. Family members argued about the funeral arrangements (different religions...we ended up having ministers from two faiths officiate). I was still ill. A family member told me she was glad Sandy was dead. I do not know how I got through it all, but I somehow muddled through, the visitation, funeral and burial in a fog.

Several women friends from church dressed Sandy for burial. This was very comforting. One of my friends purchased a beautiful white dress for her to wear.

Chapter Fourteen: My Own Special Angel

On the morning of the viewing, a Sunday after services, I fainted when I first saw my beautiful, special Sandy laying in repose in the casket. She was laid in a simple wooden box, which had been covered with an elegant, white, flowered cloth. Hundreds of people streamed through the mortuary to comfort me; friends, relatives, neighbors, her teachers and representatives, church members (The doctor who let her die dared to make an appearance; crying!). I was there from morning through the evening greeting them all. I could not leave her. When it was time to leave, Tammy, Jeff and I knelt down beside her and prayed for a few minutes. I finally had to be pulled away by family members.

The following morning, I arrived at the church just as Sandy arrived in a gray hearse. My knees buckled as her casket was rolled passed me. The church was filled with lovely, colorful and fragrant, flower arrangements. For the hour before the service, more people streamed in offering comfort, while I again stood next to Sandy in her casket. By the time the services began, the church was totally occupied. The service was consoling, yet I sat literally numb through the hour. A children's choir sang sounding like angels. I knew that Sandy was now my very own "special angel."

My knees buckled once more and I shook as my brother held me while the casket was closed for the final time. Sandy was carried out by family members, led by her "favorite grandpa," my father.

The cemetery was more than an hour away. It was a long, very long, ride. Saying my final farewell and driving away, were two of the most difficult things I have ever had to do in my life. Sandy now rests in beautiful, serene surroundings, on the side of a hill next to a small stream. (Her "favorite grandpa" is now buried close to her.) Her headstone reads, "Our Own Special Angel."

CHAPTER FIFTEEN

MY VOW

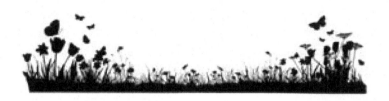

It was four months before I was finally notified that Sandy had died of overwhelming sepsis, an infection in the bloodstream; not the flu. It was also discovered that the infection showed up that night at the hospital, but no one bothered to do anything about it. The autopsy also indicated that her lungs were totally filled with fluid at the time of death; also showing up in the x-ray that night at the hospital. Indeed, Sandy had died needlessly.

About a week after the services, a friend came to visit me. She worked at the same hospital that failed us so badly. She came to tell me that when the staff and administrators discovered Sandy had passed away that night after sending us away, the hospital had a secret meeting with everyone involved and actually changed the records and got their stories straight. They knew they should never have sent her away that night.

After discussing these issues with family members, friends and lawyers, I decided to initiate a wrongful death lawsuit against the hospital, all of the doctors, nurses and technicians that were involved that fateful night.

That decision was made, not for the money, but to protect other disabled children and their families from being treated less than human. I did not want those professionals to be able to allow another child die because he or she is not "normal."

Unfortunately, the lawsuit lasted four painful years. I could not get on with my life. I had to remember every detail constantly. Again, Sandy's memory and I were treated with little dignity. At one of the hearings, the defense attorneys for the hospital explained that Sandy was not "normal" and, therefore, she was not worth as much as a normal child, monetarily. They also described her as "grotesque," having had a large brain syndrome. We immediately showed pictures to the judge and attorneys of her beautiful, smiling face.

I could not take the pressure any longer and was forced to settle out-of-court. The doctors were never punished or reprimanded. It seemed to be all for nothing. But I could not let Sandy live and die for no reason. I had to give her life and death purpose.

I vowed, then and there, that children with disabilities would never be treated without dignity if I had anything to do with it. I wanted to change things somehow. I was going to make things better for these children and their families.

I find myself back in the present in 1987. I am still unable to speak. A discussion has ensued among the other participants after the mother's emotional outburst. I am relieved as I hear my supervisor sympathetically tell the mother that we understand her frustration and we will place the boy back in her home and we will also provide some services to assist her. It is not much but it is a beginning!

CHAPTER SIXTEEN

SANDY LIVES ON

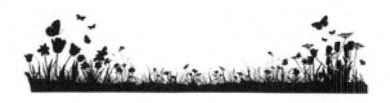

In October of 1976 I moved with my family to Sandy, Utah. In the interim I had remarried and had another daughter, Sharon Rebecca (Shari). She was a normal, healthy and happy baby. My new husband had an opportunity to become the regional manager of an airfreight company in Salt Lake City, Utah. We jumped at the chance to leave the Los Angeles, California area.

We bought a beautiful home nestled in a rural community near the entrance to one of the canyons in the Wasatch Mountains. We had a view of the entire Salt Lake Valley from our balcony. The small amount of money I received from Sandy's lawsuit was used for the down payment. I felt that the best thing I could do with the money was to invest it in a home for the family.

When Shari was old enough to go to school, I began to think about the vow I had made. I made inquiries about possible positions in the area working with disabled children. I discovered that only a few miles away a school existed for disabled children, much like the one that Sandy had attended. I was able to acquire a part time job as an aide on a wheelchair school bus.

I loved the job. The bus driver was a wonderful, caring man and the kids were great. When dropping the students off and picking them up we would wheel the students through the school: to and from their various classes. I loved what I saw. The children and teachers and staff were like one big happy family. I decided I wanted to be a part of this family.

I talked with the principal about the possibility of working in the school in some capacity. He explained that each class had a certified teacher and several aides, called training specialists, working together as a team. Only a high school diploma was needed to be a training specialist and training was done on the job. I knew this was what I wanted to do.

In only a few months a position came open and I was hired as a full time training specialist. I loved the job. The teacher was so much fun and the students were wonderful. I loved the team. I enjoyed my job so much that I actually felt guilty accepting pay.

I worked there for several years in different classes and with different teams; with children of different ages and disabling conditions. Most of the children had multiple conditions (physically and mentally disabled) and each child was unique. I learned so much about teaching and training disabled students.

After several years, my marriage fell apart. My husband had one affair after another and then I discovered that he had sexually abused my daughters. I had to leave my beloved job and students and my beautiful home and hide my daughters from this very sick individual. The State of Utah was attempting to give my children to this man who had abused them. I could not let this happen. In the process, I lost my home. He was able to convince the courts that he had used his own money to buy the house so it was given to him!! I lost everything trying to protect my children. (This is another book to write!)

Chapter Sixteen: Sandy Lives On

During the years I fought the State of Utah; with my knowledge, skills and training; I was able to readily acquire jobs working in school districts and in severely disabled adult programs in different states. I had new titles to add to my resume: teacher aide, program manager and behavior specialist. I worked with more individuals of different ages and disabling conditions and received more training along the way.

Sadly, through those years, I saw many injustices and abuses to and about the disabled children and adults and their families with which I worked. I had always been an advocate for their rights and many times I have felt the wrath of the establishment because I dared to speak out. I knew that in my positions, without a college degree, I could not make much of a difference. I felt I was not doing enough and could not stand by watching the abuses. I decided that I could do more to keep my vow if I became a certified special education teacher.

After returning to Salt Lake City, meeting Calvin Hunter, my present husband and best friend, and successfully protecting my children: at the age of 34, I began to attend classes at the University of Utah. I also returned as a training specialist to the school in which I originally began my career. I worked full time there and took full time classes while keeping a grade point average above 3.5. I had to do this in order to keep my grants and scholarships.

After several years of this grueling schedule, I decided to quit working full time. I hated to leave my students but felt with the scholarships and loans and a part time position, I could devote more time to my studies and family.

I answered an ad for a part time position as a consultant to the State of Utah, Division of Services to the Handicapped (a state level division). I never believed that I would be hired, but thought I would take a chance anyway. When they saw my resume with all of my training and skills and knew I was attending the University of Utah, they offered me the position. I was so surprised and happy!!! It was a perfect position for me. I could make my own hours around my classes and family.

At that time, normalization and deinstitutionalization were occurring all over the country due to federal mandates. Children and adults were being removed from the horrible and archaic institutions. They were being placed with families throughout the nearby communities. It was my job to go to these homes and develop the programs for the individuals being moved and train the foster parents and trainers how to work with the individuals and then provide follow-up with weekly visits.

After several months, my supervisors saw my work and how well the families were doing and offered me a full time position as the program coordinator for the program. I decided to take the position. This State Division (team) had been given the job, as dictated by the federal government, to move the children out of the Utah Training School, but no one knew what to do. When I came along, with all of my training and knowing how to develop programs, they knew I had the skills to make the plan a success.

It was the opportunity of a lifetime for me. I could be in a position to really make a difference. I now was an administrator on a state level and became a member of the Human Rights Committee. I was in a position to see that the laws protecting disabled individuals were obeyed and that the rights of disabled individuals were not violated. I was given my own office in the State Building and the use of a State car in my travels.

Luckily, I was at a point in my education where, I was able to handle the job, my studies and my family life with some good organization on my part. The Special Education Department at the University made me an adjunct professor when they discovered the position I held. Some of the professors asked me to teach some classes for them or come to some of their classes as a guest speaker, but I could never fit it into my schedule, unfortunately.

I loved what I was doing. I could not have been happier with how my life was progressing. I loved my job, my studies and my family time, but life changes; things are never static. The funding ran out for the program I was coordinating, at the same time I needed to begin my classroom practicum (experiences, on the job training for college credit) and my student teaching. It all worked out for the best, but I have always missed that State position. I have never made as much of a difference for disabled individuals as I did in that position.

I finally completed my studies and in 1988, at the age of forty. I graduated Cum Laude (3.7 grade point average) from the University of Utah, with a Bachelor of Science Degree in Special Education and a Bachelor of Science Degree in Psychology. I have teaching certificates for the Sates of Utah and Wyoming and have taught in both States. I have also consulted for the movement of individuals being removed from the institutions of Wyoming, the last state to comply with the federal laws.

Sotos Syndrome: A Tribute To Sandy

After receiving my degrees, Calvin and I moved to small town in Wyoming near the Uinta Mountains of Utah. A few years before, we bought a beautiful piece of land close to the border of Wyoming. We built a home on the property ourselves with some help from the kids over several years time. The town was the closest place for us to work and be able to continue building on our home. I taught in the school district there and then at the Wyoming State Hospital. Several years passed as our mountain home was built and I taught. Calvin was also working in the school district as he continued to drive back and forth several evenings a week (120 miles) to the University of Utah for classes. He was completing his Master of Education Degree in Special Education.

For his final year, we decided to move back to Salt Lake City to make it easier for him. (All of our children were gone by now, they all went into the military after graduation from high school.) I took a teaching position in Salt Lake City, and we leased an apartment near the University. We really missed our mountain home and the small town life in Wyoming. We went home to the mountains as often as we could.

Upon returning home, teaching positions were not available in our small Wyoming town. I accepted a position as the Program Services Director for an adult program for dual-diagnosed (intellectual disabilities and mentally ill and some were also physically disabled) individuals. I was the supervisor of 50 staff members and 100 clients. I developed their programs and trained the staff.

As much as I enjoyed this position, it was very taxing on me. I could not keep up with the demands of my job. I had to give it up. I was beginning to have some

80

serious medical concerns. I was diagnosed with Fibromyalgia at that point.

I went back to teaching when a position opened in the district. I taught on the high school level for three more years. But, as each year progressed, I became weaker and weaker and developed more and more serious symptoms. I was losing my balance, having memory problems, experiencing perceptual problems and confusion, and my arms and legs were numb and tingly at times. Walking up stairs caused horrible pain in my legs. The fatigue I experienced was nearly incapacitating. I was diagnosed with mitral valve prolapse of the heart, and degenerative disc disease of the spine. After seeing a neurologist, he thought I might have Multiple Sclerosis (MS) also.

I had to, reluctantly and with a heavy heart, give up my teaching career.

Over the last 3 years I have continued to decline. I now have a final diagnosis of MS: demyelinization of the nerves of the central nervous system. I am now disabled. I need to walk with a cane and, at times, now need a wheelchair; the pain and weakness wax and wane but never go away completely. Sitting at a computer is extremely painful for me for any length of time. I have pain in my back; neck and shoulders and my arms, hands, fingers and legs go numb after a few minutes.

Due to my declining health, I felt as if I had to give up my vow of making a difference in the lives of individuals with disabilities. It was very difficult for me to accept, especially since in every position I held, I continued to see injustices, abuses and the breaking of federal law in relationship to disabled children and adults. (It also continued as my husband taught special education after my retirement. He left his teaching career due to it. Another book in the making!) However, Calvin reminded me about my book and that if it could be published, Sandy would still live on and could make a difference for disabled individuals and their families, especially those with Sotos Syndrome. He suggested completing it and publishing it for me. I suggested adding a chapter with information about Sotos Syndrome; a resource for families. And now, with his assistance, Sandy's book has become a reality!!

I believe that Sandy did not live or die in vain. The five short years that she shared with me were not easy, nor were they always happy; but I would not choose to change them. Some of the cruel and sad things that took place have made me the person I am today. After her death and because of her life; I became an aide, training specialist, behavior specialist, teacher, consultant and program director. In each position, I made a difference, or attempted to make a difference, in the lives of the disabled children and adults entrusted to my care. Whenever and wherever I saw injustice, abuse and breaking of the law, I stepped in to correct the wrongs. I was always a student-client-parent advocate in Sandy's name.

Although I am not able to teach or consult or direct any longer, on behalf of disabled children and adults, Sandy lives on in this book and she and I can continue to make a difference.

2013

Much can happen in ten years. My diagnosis for Multiple Sclerosis (MS) turned out to be a very rare, debilitating, hereditary and difficult to diagnose disease, much like Sotos Syndrome, but I was 62 when I was finally diagnosed, 3 years ago. Periodic Paralysis is a mineral metabolic disorder called an ion channelopathy. It is often misdiagnosed and mistreated, thus causing more damage or possible death to the person with it. There are several types and the form I have, a variant of Andersen-Tawil Syndrome, is the most rare and the most serious type with approximately 1 in 60,000,000 people born with it.

On a cellular level, triggered by things such as sleep, exercise, sugar, salt, most medications, stress, cold, heat, anesthesia, adrenaline, IVs, etc., potassium wrongly enters the muscles either temporarily weakening or paralyzing the individual. Episodes can be full body lasting hours or days. Permanent muscle weakness may occur over time. If it affects the breathing muscles it can become terminal. Dangerous heart arrhythmia, heart rate fluctuation, blood pressure fluctuation, choking, breathing difficulties, cardiac arrest and/or respiratory arrest can also accompany the episodes. Due to these complications, it is extremely important to avoid the episodes. Gradual, progressive, muscular weakness can also affect the individual with this condition.

There are no known cures, but there are treatments and drugs for some forms, which can be and are successful for some individuals.

The type I have, however, has no traditional medications, which can elevate the symptoms, but by avoiding the triggers and by using some natural methods, the number of paralytic episodes can be reduced and the severity of the episodes can be lessened. Due to many wrong diagnoses and improper medications, I am now severely disabled in a power wheelchair and on oxygen therapy 24/7. I was having episodes 4 to 5 times a day but now, with the natural methods have been able to reduce the number to about 1 or 2 a month with less severity and for shorter periods of time.

Despite my illness and disability, Calvin and I are co-founders of the Periodic Paralysis Network. We have a website www.periodicparalysisnetwork.com with a forum containing 3 distinct discussion groups and a blog and recently we published a book, *living With Periodic Paralysis: The Mystery Unraveled*, which is an extension of our website and the only book written about this condition. We work towards the improvement of the quality and safety of patients from all over the world with the various forms of Periodic Paralysis. Our focus is on educational resources to build self-reliance and self-empowerment and to prevent possible harm from improper treatment. Our approach to treatment focuses on the self-monitoring of vitals and the management of symptoms through natural methods. We also offer strategies to understanding the disease, getting a proper diagnosis, managing the symptoms, and assisting caregivers and family members. We get new members almost daily from all over the world (Iran, Ukraine, Turkey, Denmark, Wales, Netherlands, Canada, Finland, Australia, Argentina, Pakistan, Bangladesh, Philippines and more) that are seeking help for themselves, their children and entire families and are unable to find it anywhere. We provide ideas on how to find doctors, get a diagnosis, get the proper help in the ER, how to discover their triggers and more.

I am not able to teach, consult or direct in the traditional ways any longer, however, I do continue to teach, consult and direct and much more with the help of modern technology. Sandy lives on in this book and in my continuing work with disabled children and adults with Periodic Paralysis. She and I can continue to make a difference.

Sandy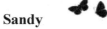

Oh Sandy, dear Sandy, my Sandy;
Where are you?
Where are you now?
Where is your sweet little face?
Slightly misshapen, but nevertheless beautiful?
Or those cute little dimples, and constantly flushed cheeks?
Where are those freckles?
Or your turned up nose?
And what of your long flowing hair?
Do the auburn curls still frame your pale little face?
Where are your twinkling blue eyes, filled with mischief?
Yet filled with a certain sadness and longing?
Are they closed forever?
Where is that never-ending smile that was always such a comfort?
And your laugh, your sweet little giggle, unmistakably yours?
Is it silenced forever in the stillness of Eternity?
What of your poor defenseless body?
Does it still carry the wretched scars of the
Injustices dealt you during your short five years of life?
Do you walk with the same awkward gait unique only to you?
Or has Providence straightened your crooked little limbs?
Do you run and jump now?
Do you play with other children?
Or do you continue to sleep in the darkness of time?
I think not, Sandy.
You are very much alive.

For you live on in my heart and memory and will for an eternity.

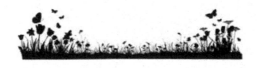

CHAPTER SEVENTEEN

PHOTO ALBUM

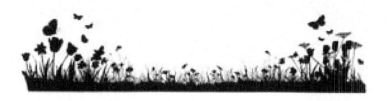

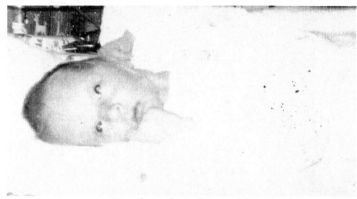

Sandy a few days old.

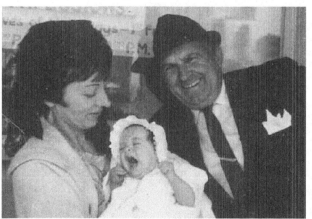

Six weeks old, baptism day with Knittle grandparents.

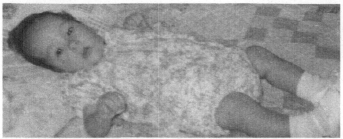

Four months old. First Easter. Curved leg.

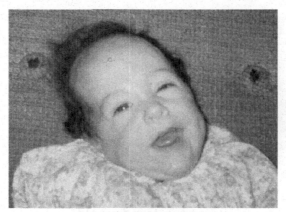

Weak neck muscles.

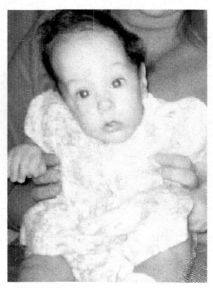

High forehead.

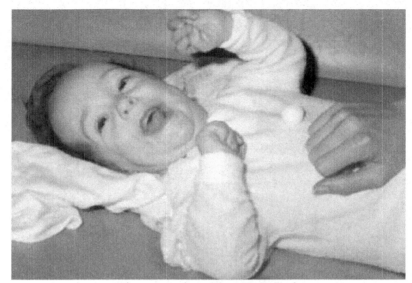

Five months old at Fort Ord.

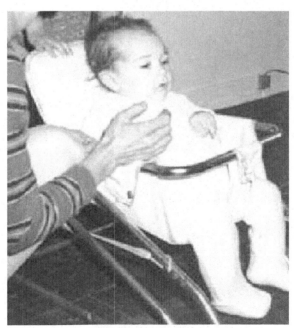

Sandy at Fort Ord.

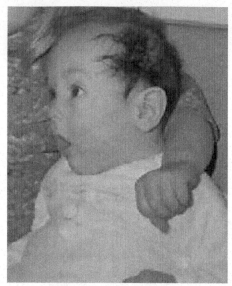

Sandy at Fort Ord

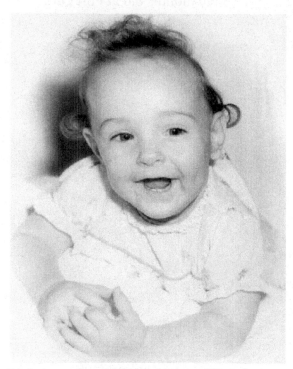

Eight months old in body cast. Dimples.

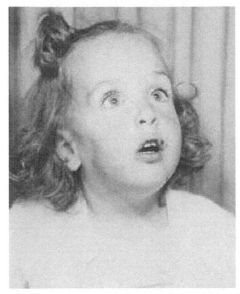

At the county fair. About 20 months old.

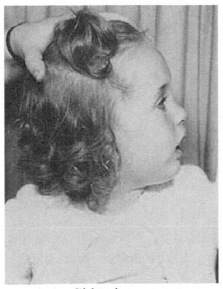

Side view.

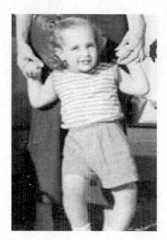

Finally standing

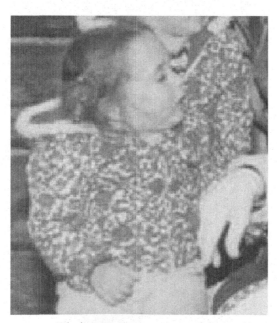

Christmas two years old.

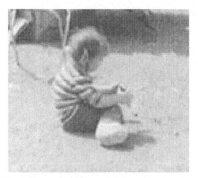

At family picnic with casts on legs.

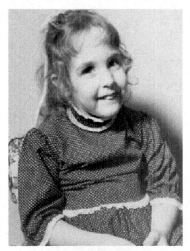

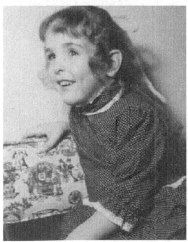

Christmas 3 years old.

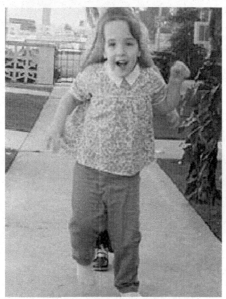

Running. Three years old.

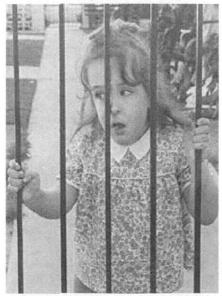

Looking thru gate. Gum in mouth.

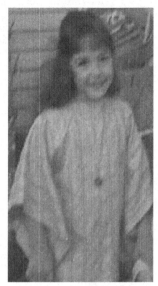

Angel dresses, three years old.

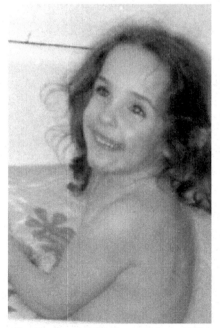

In the bathtub three years old

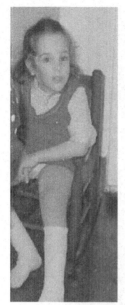 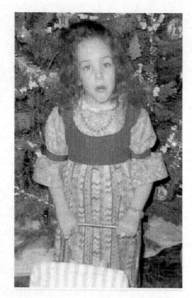

After the cast.   Christmas four years old.
Candy in mouth

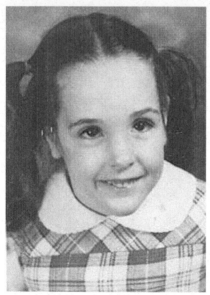

School picture four years old.

CHAPTER EIGHTEEN

ABOUT SOTOS SYNDROME

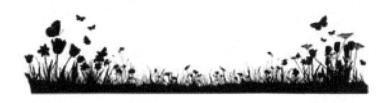

Sotos Syndrome, is a little known and very rare, genetic, overgrowth disorder; which is clearly evidenced by accelerated physical growth; abnormally large hands and feet; distinctive face and head features, narrow and highly arched palate, mental and developmental delays and poor muscle tone and coordination. The syndrome was first described in the New England Journal of Medicine in 1964. According to research, in 1994, there were fewer than 200 known instances of it in the world. Statistics indicate that now one in about fourteen thousand children are born with Sotos syndrome, but due to the difficulty in diagnosing and lack of reporting, it is thought that actually one in five-thousand children is born with Sotos. It is not life threatening and individuals with it may live a normal life span. No established method of treatment exists for the syndrome; treatment is administered based on the symptoms that occur. [1, 2, 3, 4, 5, 6, 7]

Typically, a baby born with Sotos Syndrome is larger than normal. The fast growth pattern continues into the fourth to fifth year of life, at which time it tends to normalize. The growing ceases normally, however, at puberty. A four-year-old child may have the height and weight of a child of eight or nine years and, thus, the term "gigantism". X-rays reveal advanced maturation of the bones for the age of the child. Into adulthood, a male may reach 6' 8", a female 6' 2". [1, 2, 4, 5, 6]

Individuals with Sotos have heads that are larger, longer and narrower than normal. Their foreheads project outward minimally and are wider with a higher than normal hairline. They usually have tapering chins. Eyes are set far apart and are down sloping at the outside corners. When the mouth is closed, the upper and lower sets of teeth do not come together due to a difference in the length of the jaws. [1, 2, 3, 4, 5, 6]

Hands are abnormally large with a "chubby" appearance. The feet are also extremely large. It is not uncommon to see an adult with Sotos wear a size 18 shoes. Fallen arches and weak ankles are common problems. The arm span is larger than a person's height. [5, 7]

Those with this syndrome stand bending forward, to a small degree, with their head protruding slightly and bending knees. An awkward, unique way of walking and clumsiness are present due to poor gross motor skills and poor muscle tone throughout the body. [1, 3, 4, 5]

Typically, an individual is intellectually challenged with the average IQ 72, which is considered low normal or mildly intellectually challenged. The child may require special education. An individual with Sotos, however, may have a normal IQ. [1, 3, 4, 5, 6, 7]

The roof of the mouth is very high and narrow at birth. This combined with poor muscle tone and the problem of the jaws not meeting, cause feeding and sucking problems as an infant. As an older child, eating, chewing and speech problems result. Drooling and breathing through the mouth are also problematic. [1, 2, 3, 4, 5, 6, 7]

Developmentally, delays may be present in all areas; fine (using fingers and hands) and gross (walking, balance) motor, cognition (understanding), social, emotional, speech and toilet training. However, receptive language, or the understanding of what is said, is more accelerated than the expressive or conveyance of ideas. In other words, they are able to understand what to say, long before they are able to say it, thus creating frustration for the child. [1, 2, 3, 4, 5, 6, 7]

Behaviorally, many different patterns may develop: aggression, quickness to anger, easy annoyance, excessive fears or dread, unwanted compulsive ideas or emotions, dislike for change in routine, short attention span, hyperactivity, withdrawal, no-communication, or repetitive actions. [1, 2, 3]

Other features, which may be seen in an individual with Sotos Syndrome, include:

Curvature of the spine
Teeth coming in earlier than normal
Clubfeet, deformed and dislocated hip sockets
Lack of sensitivity to pain, heat or cold
Risk for tumors and some cancers
Scalp sensitivity
Recurring ear infections
Recurring upper respiratory illnesses
High fevers when ill
Seizures due to high fevers
Loose ligaments (floppy)
Flushed (red and warm) cheeks
Slightly enlarged ventricles (cavities which carry fluids) in the brain
Allergies
Asthma
Constipation

Narrowing where the sigmoid colon and rectum meet, causing enlargement of the bowel.

Enlargement of the area beneath the membrane that covers the brain

Rapid and rhythmic movement of the eyeball from side to side

Non-alignment of the eyes (crossed-eyes)

Increased perspiration

Over or under activity of the thyroid [1, 2, 3, 4, 5, 6, 7]

(It has been noted that most challenges of this disorder improve with age.[4])

Sotos is not a syndrome that is easily and quickly diagnosed at birth. It may take several years of testing, observation and misdiagnoses before a definite and final diagnosis can be reached.

No cure for Sotos Syndrome exists. Treatment is aimed at relieving the symptoms that occur, rather than to eliminate the cause, because it is not possible. [1, 3]

Due to the many developmental delays experienced with this condition; the sooner treatment, training, therapy and education can begin, the better the final results will be for the child and family. [3,]

Sotos Syndrome: A Cause?

In April of 2002, a genetics research group, N. Kurotaki, et al, in Nagasaki, Japan, announced they discovered a gene they believe to be related to the cause of Sotos Syndrome. The report was published in Nature Genetics 30:365-366. They believe "haploinsufficiency" of the NSD1 gene at chromosome

5 is the cause. This term means a rearrangement, malfunction or deletion of the gene. It is now known that the NSD1 gene is specifically at chromosome 5q35 and about 75% of the known cases are due to this mutation. NSD1 is responsible for making the protein used in normal development and growth. About 95% of the cases of Sotos Syndrome have no known family history of the condition. [1, 2, 3, 7, 8, 9]

Typing "Sotos Syndrome", into any search engine, can find the latest information about this condition on the Internet. There are websites, support groups, medical journal articles, Facebook pages, handbooks, You Tube videos and much more available for families, caregivers, social workers, teachers and doctors to learn more or connect with others. The "Works Cited" at the end of this chapter has great sources for information as well as many more references at each site.

Works Cited:

1. Wikipedia. (September 2013). Sotos syndrome. Retrieved from: http://en.wikipedia.org/wiki/Sotos_syndrome

2. U.S. National Library of Medicine. Genetics Home Reference. (November 2013). Sotos syndrome. Retrieved from: http://ghr.nlm.nih.gov/condition/sotos-syndrome

3. Orphanet Journal of Rare Diseases. (September 2017). Sotos syndrome. Retrieved from: http://www.ojrd.com/content/2/1/36

4. Sotos Syndrome Support Association. (2005). What is Sotos Syndrome. Retrieved from: http://sotossyndrome.org/sotos-syndrome

5. Child Growth Foundation. (2012). Sotos Syndrome. Retrieved from: http://www.childgrowthfoundation.org/Default.aspx?page=Conditionssot os

6. Child Growth Foundation. (2012). Sotos Syndrome-parents guide. Retrieved from: http://www.childgrowthfoundation.org/CMS/FILES/Sotos_Syndrome_- _parents_guide.pdf

7. MD Consult. (2011). Kliegman: Nelson Textbook of Pediatrics, 19th ed. Sotos Syndrome (Cerebral Gigantism). Retrieved from: http://www.mdconsult.com/books/page.do?eid=4-u1.0-B978-1-4377- 0755-7..00554-6--f0010&isbn=978-1-4377-0755- 7&type=bookPage&from=content&uniqId=431758412-2

8. OMIM (Online Mendelian Inheritance in Man). (May 2013). SOTOS SYNDROME 1; SOTOS1. Retrieved from: http://omim.org/entry/117550

9. PubMed Health. (2002). Haploinsuffiency of NSD1 Causes Sotos syndrome. Retrieved from: http://www.ncbi.nlm.nih.gov/pubmed/11896389?dopt=Abstract&holding =f1000,f1000m,isrctn

About the Authors

Susan Quentine Knittle-Hunter had a daughter, Sandra Renissa, who was born with Sotos Syndrome. Sandy lived to be only five years old. But, during those five short years, Susan learned much about the weaknesses, which existed in the medical, educational and social aspects of the life for children with disabilities and their families. After Sandy's death, Susan made a vow to spend the rest of her life working to improve the quality of life for disabled children and adults. She attended the University of Utah and graduated with a B.S. in Special Education and a B.S. in Psychology. She has taught children of all ages and disabling conditions in Utah and Wyoming. She has been a consultant on the state level for the States of Utah and Wyoming working with disabled children and adults and their families. Susan has designed several community adult living programs. She has written an instructional manual, *Creating Program Plans for MR/DD Adults,* and has presented workshops using the manual. She was a program coordinator for an adult habilitation program in Wyoming. Susan became disabled herself with Periodic Paralysis and had to give up her career devoted to improving the lives of challenged children and adults.

Calvin Hunter has two B.S. Degrees in Behavioral Science and Psychology and a Masters Degree in Special Education. He has been a resource teacher teaching middle school age learning and behavior challenged students. He has written a book about his experiences building their home in the Uinta Mountains in Utah.

Together they wrote the first edition of this book and published it as an eBook in 2003 and have now completed the second edition.

Presently, they have just completed writing and publishing *living with Periodic Paralysis: The Mystery Unraveled.* Over 400 pages, it answers all of the questions of the what, when, where, how and why of Periodic Paralysis and unravels all of the mysteries of this rare condition. Despite both being ill, they continue to help individuals with Periodic Paralysis through the organization they co-founded the Periodic Paralysis Network. They have a website and a forum containing 3 distinct discussion groups including a support and education group and a blog where they continue to teach daily.

Calvin and Susan, married for over 32 years, enjoy the peace and beauty of the forest in their new home in Sequim, Washington. They live with their two spoiled cats and plenty of wildlife. They are presently writing their next books and continue to work daily to help others with PP. In their spare time, Calvin enjoys working with wood and tends their organic garden while Susan enjoys genealogy research and reading historical romance novels.

CPSIA information can be obtained
at www.ICGtesting.com
Printed in the USA
LVOW01s2145160816
500619LV00019BA/1036/P